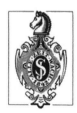

Progress in Pediatric Surgery

Volume 24

Cofounding Editor
P. P. Rickham

Editors
T. A. Angerpointner, Munich
M. W. L. Gauderer · W. Ch. Hecker
J. Prévot · L. Spitz
U. G. Stauffer · P. Wurnig

Constipation and Fecal Incontinence and Motility Disturbances of the Gut

Volume Editors
J. Yokoyama, Tokyo
T. A. Angerpointner, Munich

With 113 Figures and 62 Tables

Springer-Verlag Berlin Heidelberg New York
London Paris Tokyo Hong Kong

Professor JOTARO YOKOYAMA, MD
Assistant Professor of Pediatric Surgery
School of Medicine, Keio University
35 Shinanomachi Shinjuku-ku
Tokyo, Japan

Priv.-Doz. Dr. THOMAS A. ANGERPOINTNER
Zenettistraße 48/III, D-8000 Munich 2
Federal Republic of Germany

Volumes 1–17 of this series were published
by Urban & Schwarzenberg, Baltimore–Munich

ISBN-13:978-3-642-74495-2   e-ISBN-13:978-3-642-74493-8
DOI: 10.1007/978-3-642-74493-8

Library of Congress Cataloging-in-Publication Data
Constipation and fecal incontinence and motility disturbances of the gut /
volume editors, J. Yokoyama, Th. A. Angerpointner.
  p. cm. – (Progress in pediatric surgery; v. 24)
Includes bibliographical references.
ISBN-13:978-3-642-74495-2 (U.S.: alk. paper)
1. Constipation in children. 2. Fecal incontinence in children. 3. Gastrointestinal motility disorders in children. I. Yokoyama, J. (Jotaro), 1936– . II. Angerpointner, Thomas. III. Series.
[DNLM: 1. Constipation – in infancy. 2. Fecal Incontinence – in infancy & childhood. 3. Gastrointestinal Diseases – in infancy & childhood. 4. Gastrointestinal Motility – in infancy & childhood.
W1 PR677KA v. 24 / WS 310 C758]   RD137.A1P7 vol. 24   [RJ456.C76]   617.9'8 s – dc20
[618.92'33]   DNLM/DLC   89-21805

This work is subject to copyright. All rights are reserved, whether the whole or part of the material is concerned, specifically the rights of translation, reprinting, reuse of illustrations, recitation, broadcasting, reproduction on microfilms or in other ways, and storage in data banks. Duplication of this publication or parts thereof is only permitted under the provisions of the German Copyright Law of September 9, 1965, in its version of June 24, 1985, and a copyright fee must always be paid. Violations fall under the prosecution act of the German Copyright Law.

© Springer-Verlag Berlin Heidelberg 1989
Softcover reprint of the hardcover 1st edition 1989

The use of registered names, trademarks, etc. in this publication does not imply, even in the absence of a specific statement, that such names are exempt from the relevant protective laws and regulations and therefore free for general use.

Product liability: The publisher can give no guarantee for information about drug dosage and application thereof contained in this book. In every individual case the respective user must check its accuracy by consulting other pharmaceutical literature.

2123/3145-543210   Printed on acid-free paper

Table of Contents

Part I: Constipation and Fecal Incontinence

Preface. M. KASAI 3

Studies on the Rectoanal Reflex in Children and in Experimental Animals: An Evaluation of Neuronal Control of the Rectoanal Reflex. J. YOKOYAMA, S. NAMBA, N. IHARA, H. MATSUFUGI, T. KURODA, S. HIROBE, K. KATSUMATA, K. TAMURA, and H. TAKAHIRA. With 11 Figures 5

Computerized Analysis of Anorectal Manometry. M. SAKANIWA, S. SAWAGUCHI, H. OHKAWA, and K. IKEBUKURO. With 11 Figures . . 21

The Electromyographic Examination to Evaluate the External Sphincter Muscle in Anorectal Malformations. A. HAYASHI, J. YOKOYAMA, and K. KATSUMATA. With 4 Figures . . 33

Diagnosis of Hirschsprung's Disease by Anorectal Manometry. A. NAGASAKI, K. SUMITOMO, T. SHONO, and K. IKEDA. With 5 Figures 40

Problems in Diagnosis of Hirschsprung's Disease by Anorectal Manometry. J. YOKOYAMA, T. KURODA, H. MATSUFUGI, S. HIROBE, S. HARA, and K. KATSUMATA. With 5 Figures 49

Anorectal Manometry After Ikeda's Z-Shaped Anastomosis in Hirschsprung's Disease. A. NAGASAKI, K. SUMITOMO, T. SHONO, and K. IKEDA. With 3 Figures 59

Motility of the Anorectum After the Soave-Denda Operation. Y. MORIKAWA, H. MATSUFUGI, S. HIROBE, J. YOKOYAMA, and K. KATSUMATA. With 3 Figures 67

Anorectal Motility After Rectal Myectomy in Patients with Hirschsprung's Disease. R. OHI and K. KOMATSU. With 3 Figures 77

Continence and Reflex Pressure Profile After Surgery to Correct the Imperforate Anus. M. ISHIHARA and K. MORITA. With 4 Figures 86

Management of Defecation in Spina Bifida. M. MAIE, M. SAKANIWA,
H. TAKAHASHI, and J. IWAI. With 2 Figures 97

Anorectal Motility in Children with Complete Rectal Prolapse.
H. SUZUKI, S. AMANO, K. MATSUMOTO, and Y. TSUKAMOTO.
With 8 Figures 105

Rectoanal Pressure Studies and Postoperative Continence
in Imperforate Anus.
N. IWAI, J. YANAGIHARA, K. TOKIWA, and T. TAKAHASHI 115

Part II: Motility Disturbances of the Gut

Preface. T. A. ANGERPOINTNER 123

Electrophysiological Principles of Motility Disturbances in the
Small and Large Intestines — Review of the Literature
and Personal Experience. A. M. HOLSCHNEIDER. With 10 Figures . 125

The Practical Significance of Manometry in Pathology of the
Rectum and Anorectum. A. F. SCHÄRLI. With 11 Figures 142

Functional Colonic Ultrasonography: Normal Findings of Colonic
Motility and Follow-Up in Neuronal Intestinal Dysplasia. G. PISTOR.
With 13 Figures 155

The Influence of Small Bowel Contamination on the Pathogenesis of
Bowel Obstruction. M. SCHWÖBEL, J. HIRSIG, O. ILLI, and U. BÄTTIG.
With 4 Figures 165

Diagnosis of Innervation-Related Motility Disorders of the Gut
and Basic Aspects of Enteric Nervous System Development.
J. C. MOLENAAR, D. TIBBOEL, A. W. M. VAN DER KAMP,
and J. H. C. MEIJERS. With 1 Figure 173

Neuronal Intestinal Dysplasia. R. RINTALA, J. RAPOLA, and I. LOUHIMO.
With 2 Figures 186

Motility Malfunction of the Gastrointestinal Tract
by Rare Diseases — Fibrosis of the Intestinal Wall.
R. DAUM, W. NÜTZENADEL, H. ROTH, and Z. ZACHARIOU.
With 6 Figures 193

Transient Functional Obstruction of the Colon in Neonates: Examination of Its Development by Manometry and Biopsies.
G. LASSMANN, A. KEES, K. KÖRNER, and P. WURNIG. With 5 Figures   202

Total Colonic Aganglionosis. G. MENARDI and J. HAGER.
With 2 Figures 217

Surgical Management of Chronic Intestinal Pseudo-obstruction in Infancy and Childhood.
E. W. FONKALSRUD, H. A. PITT, W. E. BERQUIST, and M. E. AMENT . 221

The Importance of Oral Sodium Replacement in Ileostomy Patients.
P. SACHER, J. HIRSIG, J. GRESSER, and L. SPITZ 226

Subject Index 233

List of Editors

Angerpointner, T. A., Priv.-Doz. Dr.
  Zenettistraße 48/III, D-8000 München 2

Gauderer, Michael, W. L., MD
  University Pediatric Surgical Associates, 2101 Adelbert Road
  Cleveland, OH 44106, USA

Hecker, W. Ch., Prof. Dr.
  Kinderchirurgische Klinik im Dr. von Haunerschen Kinderspital
  der Universität München, Lindwurmstraße 4
  D-8000 München 2

Prévot, J., Prof.
  Clinique Chirurgical Pédiatrique, Hôpital d'Enfants de Nancy
  F-54511 Vandœvre Cedex

Rickham, P. P., Prof. Dr.
  MD, MS, FRCS, FRCSI, FRACS, DCH, FAAP
  Universitätskinderklinik, Chirurgische Abteilung
  Steinwiesstraße 75, CH-8032 Zürich

Spitz, L., Prof., PhD, FRCS, Nuffield Professor of Pediatric Surgery
  Institute of Child Health, University of London
  Hospital for Sick Children, Great Ormond Street, 30 Guilford Street
  GB-London WC1N 1EH

Stauffer, U. G., Prof. Dr.
  Universitätskinderklinik, Kinderchirurgische Abteilung
  Steinwiesstraße 75, CH-8032 Zürich

Wurnig, P., Prof. Dr.
  Kinderchirurgische Abteilung des
  Mautner Markhof'schen Kinderspitals
  Baumgasse 75, A-1030 Wien

List of Contributors

You will find the addresses at the beginning of the respective contribution

Amano, S.   105
Ament, M. E.   221
Angerpointner, T. A.   123
Berquist, W. E.   221
Bättig, U.   165
Daum, R.   193
Fonkalsrud, E. W.   221
Gresser, J.   226
Hager, J.   217
Hara, S.   49
Hayashi, A.   33
Hirobe, S.   5, 49, 67
Hirsig, J.   165, 226
Holschneider, A. M.   125
Ihara, N.   5
Ikebukuro, K..   21
Ikeda, K.   40, 59
Illi, O.   165
Ishihara, M.   86
Iwai, J.   97
Iwai, N.   115
Kasai, M.   3
Katsumata, K.   5, 33, 49, 67
Kees, A.   202
Komatsu, K.   77
Körner, K.   202
Kuroda, T.   5, 49
Lassmann, G.   202
Louhimo, I.   186
Maie, M.   97
Matsufugi, H.   5, 49, 67
Matsumoto, K.   105
Meijers, J. H. C.   173
Menardi, G.   217
Molenaar, J. C.   173
Morikawa, Y.   67
Morita, K.   86
Nagasaki, A.   40, 59
Namba, S.   5
Nützenadel, W.   193
Ohi, R.   77
Ohkawa, H.   21
Pistor, G.   155
Pitt, I. A.   221
Rapola, J.   186
Rintala, R.   186
Roth, H.   193
Sacher, P.   226
Sakaniwa, M.   21, 97
Sawaguchi, S.   21
Schärli, A. F.   142
Schwöbel, M.   165
Shono, T.   40, 59
Spitz, L.   226
Sumitomo, K.   40, 59
Suzuki, H.   105
Takahashi, H.   97
Takahashi, T.   115
Takahira, H.   5
Tamura, K.   5
Tibboel, D.   173
Tokiwa, K.   115
Tsukamato, Y.   105
van der Kamp, A. W. M.   173
Wurnig, P.   202
Yanagihara, J.   115
Yokoyama, J.   5, 33, 49, 67
Zachariou, Z.   193

Part I
Constipation and Fecal Incontinence

Preface

The clinical application of anorectal manometry was pioneered by pediatric surgeons. Swenson in 1949 reported that the aganglionic bowel of patients with Hirschsprung's disease did not show any propulsive movements. In 1967 Lawson and Nixon and Schnaufer et al. found that the rectosphincteric reflex, which is observed in both normal individuals and patients with chronic idiopathic constipation, is absent in patients with Hirschsprung's disease, and suggested anorectal manometry to be useful for the differentiation of Hirschsprung's disease from chronic idiopathic constipation.

Studies on the pathophysiology of constipation and incontinence problems have flourished in Japan; the Japanese Research Society for Anorectal Manometry in Childhood was founded in 1975 by Ikeda, Okamoto, Katsumata, and Kasai. The Society has contributed greatly to advances in the clinical application of anorectal manometry. Basic investigations on the function of the anorectum in both normal individuals and patients with constipation or incontinence problems have also been promoted by members of the Society. The technique of anorectal manometry has been refined and standardized. The criteria for manometric diagnosis of Hirschsprung's disease have been established. And the correlation between postoperative continence in patients with Hirschsprung's disease or anorectal malformation and manometric findings has been understood.

In this section, works by members of the Society are presented.

Professor MORIO KASAI, Sendai, Japan

Studies on the Rectoanal Reflex in Children and in Experimental Animals: An Evaluation of Neuronal Control of the Rectoanal Reflex

J. Yokoyama[1], S. Namba[1], N. Ihara[1], H. Matsufugi[1], T. Kuroda[1], S. Hirobe[1], K. Katsumata[1], K. Tamura[2], and H. Takahira[2]

Summary

A single-chamber pressure probe for rectal electromanometry was developed which seems to be superior to the complicated multichamber systems not only for clinical but also for experimental purposes. Measurements of rectoanal reflex were carried out in 268 cases with abnormal bowel function, in 103 cases following operation for Hirschsprung's disease, and in 61 cases of imperforate anus to assess postoperative continence. Experimental studies were performed in 36 dogs, 27 of which were used for short-term and 9 for long-term studies. The results of clinical and experimental studies are described and discussed, with accompanying literature. From clinical and experimental studies, the neuronal pathways of the rectoanal reflex are schematized. The normal rectoanal reflex is mediated by both the sacral cord and the myenteric neurons. It is concluded that measurements of the anal resting pressure and the rectoanal reflex constitute a valuable method to distinguish between normal and pathological sacral and myenteric innervation.

Zusammenfassung

Eine Einkammerdrucksonde zur Elektromanometrie wurde entwickelt, die nicht nur für klinische, sondern auch für experimentelle Untersuchungen Vorteile gegenüber den komplizierten Mehrkammersystemen aufzuweisen scheint. Messungen des rektoanalen Reflexes wurden bei 268 Fällen mit abnormer Darmfunktion, bei 103 Fällen nach Megacolon-congenitum-Hirschsprung-Operation und bei 61 Fällen von Analatresie zur Bestimmung der postoperativen Kontinenz durchgeführt. Experimentelle Untersuchungen wurden an 36 Hunden vorgenommen, und zwar für 27 Kurzzeit- und 9 Langzeitstudien. Die Ergebnisse der klinischen und experimentellen Messungen werden dargestellt und zusammen mit Angaben aus der Literatur diskutiert. Aufgrund von klinischen und experimentellen Studien wurden die neuronalen Verbindungen des rektoanalen Reflexes dargestellt. Ein normaler rektoanaler Reflex wird sowohl durch präsakrale als auch myenterische neuronale Elemente vermittelt. Die Bestimmung des analen Ruhedrucks und des rektoanalen Reflexes ist eine verläßliche Methode, zwischen normaler und pathologischer präsakraler und myenterischer Innervation zu unterscheiden.

Résumé

Une sonde manométrique à une seule chambre pour l'électromanométrie vient d'être mise au point. Ses avantages semblent certains, tant du point de vue expérimental que clinique, par comparaison avec la sonde à chambres multiples plus compliquée. Dans 268 cas de fonction intestinale anormale, 103 cas d'intervention chirurgicale pour maladie de Hirschsprung et 61 cas d'atrésie anale, des mesures du réflexe recto-anal pour déterminer le degré de continence post-

---

[1] Department of Pediatric Surgery, School of Medicine Keio University; 35 Shinanomachi, Shinjuku-ku, Tokyo 160, Japan
[2] Department of Physiology, Tokai University School of Medicine, Boseidai Isehara 259, Japan

opératoire ont été effectuées. Les études expérimentales ont été faites sur 36 chiens. Il y a eu 27 études de courte durée et 9 études de longue durée. Les résultats des mesures cliniques et expérimentales sont présentés et discutés en fonction de la littérature disponible. Le mode de transmission de l'influx neuronal traduisant le réflexe recto-anal a été déterminé par les études cliniques et expérimentales. Un réflexe recto-anal normal est déclenché à la fois par la chorde sacrale et les neurones myentériques. La mesure de la pression anale de repos et du réflexe recto-anal est une méthode fiable permettant la distinction entre innervation normale et innervation présacrale et myentérique pathologique.

Introduction

Since the kymographic recordings by Gaston (1948) the so-called "differential" or "multichamber" manometric recordings in the anal canal have been widely used for clinical diagnosis of Hirschsprung's disease and for pathophysiological analysis of lower bowel functions. The principle of this multichamber probe was modernized with transducers and polygraphic recording systems by Schnaufer and Talbert (1967) and Lawson and Nixon (1967), and the same principle was followed with the so-called "tandem" system of multichannel side-opening catheters (Holschneider 1974; Meunier and Mollard 1977). This trend toward modernization spread among pediatric surgeons in Japan during the early 1970s.

Establishing a suitable setting for such an elaborate multichamber probe in the variable length of the anal canal, however, was quite a difficult task, especially when the measurement was required urgently for clinical reasons. Furthermore, even when appropriately "differential" recordings were obtained from multiple foci in the anal canal, these records provided little information for the diagnosis of Hirschsprung's disease; instead, they led to many arguments concerning the old controversy between external versus internal sphincter responsiveness for anal canal pressure.

In the beginning of 1970, we devised a simple "single-chamber" manometric probe. This probe was quite easy to use even in view of the variable length of the anal canal because it was aimed toward detecting any pressure change disclosed over the entire length of the anal canal. Later, several important questions arose among us: Firstly, could this nondifferential manometric probe record meaningful pressure changes without cancelling the respective alterations originating from different foci in the anal canal? Is it possible to detect the intraluminal pressure as exactly as with the small side-opening catheter? Secondly, does the presence of such an obturator with a less flexible metallic shaft itself induce any disturbance in physiological response in the anal canal? Is it still possible to record the reflex response correctly for the purpose of diagnosis and determination of the mechanism involved?

In the following section, we present a means by which many clinical cases can be diagnosed by testing with this single-chamber probe. The results of animal experiments are then given. Here we attempt to determine what kind of activity can be revealed by our single-chamber probe in comparison with simultaneous recordings of electrical activities of internal and external sphincters. The results show the stability and identity of the anal-canal response explored by our simple, single-chamber probe. From our point of view, this simple system seems to be superior to the complicated multichamber system not only for clinical purposes but also for experimental analysis.

Clinical Studies

Material and Methods

Since 1971 we have measured the rectoanal reflex in 268 cases with abnormal bowel function and in 103 cases after operation for Hirschsprung's disease to estimate objectively the continence of patients. We have also studied the rectoanal reflex in 61 cases of imperforate anus to assess objectively the postoperative continence.

Operations on 21 cases of Hirschsprung's disease in the early period (before 1963) in our series were performed by Swenson's method. After 1964, 114 cases were treated by the Soave-Denda technique[1] (Denda 1965; Nixon 1978). Six cases of the remaining 33 were treated using the Duhamel-Ikeda procedure (Ikeda 1966), 8 cases by sphincterectomy, and 6 cases of extensive aganglionosis using Martin's method; Soave's original operative procedure was performed on 13 cases.

The rectoanal reflex was measured in 61 cases of 130 imperforate anus postoperatively treated at Keio University Hospital between 1961 and 1986. Our policy as regards the operation at present involves perineal anoplasty for low types and an abdomino-extended sacroperineal approach (Yokoyama and Katsumata 1985) for intermediate and high types. However, in high-type anomalies, various operative procedures have been attempted in the past. The abdominoperineal procedure was done in 11 cases before 1966, the original Rehbein procedure in 11 cases between 1967 and 1974, and our original abdomino-extended sacroperineal procedure in 13 cases after 1975.

Apparatus for measurement of the rectoanal reflex was the stainless-steel double-lumen water-filled pressure sensor probe, invented by Yokoyama and Namba in 1971 (Fig. 1). The inner lumen is an air channel for filling the balloon to distend the rectal wall, while the outer lumen is the pressure-measuring system which is filled with water and connected to a transducer by polyethylene tubing. The advantage of this probe is the sensitive pressure detector, with a 13-mm length for newborns and a 15-mm length for infants located at the tip of the probe. The sensitive detector is a 50-micron polyurethane membrane with particular elasticity to detect tiny pressure changes in the anal canal (Ito and Yokoyama 1981).

---

[1] This method originated with Prof. T. Denda in our University. The colon is pulled through the muscular cylinder of the rectum similarly as in the Soave method. However, primary anastomosis between this pulled-through colon and the inverted mucosa of the rectoanus is performed at the level of 2 cm oral to the mucocutaneous junction. This point differs from that in Soave's original method. Three years after our report (Denda 1965), a similar method was reported elsewhere (Boley et al. 1968).

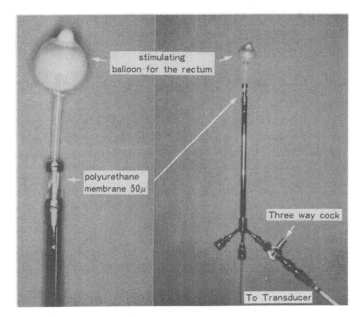
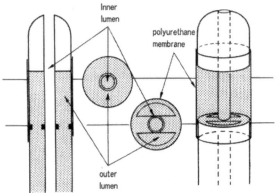

Fig. 1. Our original measuring system, K-Y probe of rectoanal reflex

The patient is laid in Sims' position. A balloon for distension is inserted into the rectum, and the membrane portion of the probe is set in the anal canal as shown in Fig. 2.

The volume of water in the measuring system must be adjusted via the three-way cock to result in approximately 30–50 cm H_2O resting pressure at the anal canal. The pressure sensor membrane should not be overdistended.

For measurement of the rectoanal reflex, rectal distension by the balloon is done four times; for the initial three times, the rectum is distended for 2–3 s, and for the last one, the duration of distension is prolonged. Following each distension, a 2- to 3-s delay is recorded before the pressure starts to fall. The pressure

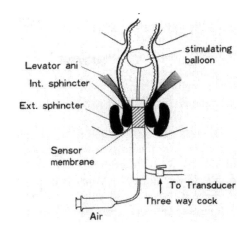

Fig. 2. Insertion of the rectal stimulating balloon into the rectum and the membrane portion of the probe in the anal canal

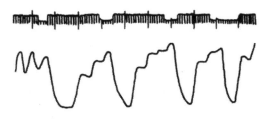

Fig. 3. A typical rectoanal reflex *(upper trace)* and the lack of reflex response in Hirschsprung's disease *(lower trace)*. *Uppermost lines* of each trace indicate the time mark of durations of distended balloon

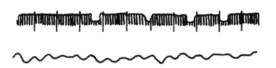

returns to baseline usually after 10–13 s in normal cases. Even if the distension is prolonged, i.e., if the balloon is kept inflated, the pressure returns to baseline as in the ordinary response. We think that the presence of the time delay before the pressure fall and the return to baseline under prolonged distension rule out any mechanical artifact which might be produced by inflation of the balloon (Fig. 3). If we obtain typical responses by the four successive distensions, we interpret the data to indicate that the patient has normal responsiveness of the rectoanal reflex; in other word, the mechanism of the rectoanal reflex is intact.

Results of Clinical Studies

Rectoanal Reflex in Cases with Abnormal Bowel Function. We measured the rectoanal reflex in 268 cases with abnormal bowel function. Among these cases,

157 exhibited typical reflex responses, and Hirschsprung's disease was thus ruled out. The other 111 cases showed no evident reflex response; in 33 of these cases the reflex response was equivocal at the initial examination. We therefore repeated the test two or three times and finally concluded that the reflex response was actually lacking. In 95 of the 111 cases with an undetectable reflex response, aganglionic bowels were confirmed by histochemical examination or histological studies.

The six cases of premature babies who lacked a detectable rectoanal reflex at the initial examination, however, showed the normal reflex 2-3 weeks after the initial test. Aside from the premature babies, ten other cases showed unexpected results. These did not demonstrate an ordinary reflex response in spite of the non-aganglionic bowels evidenced by histological studies. In the cases with sepsis, the resting anal-canal pressure showed an extremely low value, and the low anal-canal pressure might have been responsible for the undetectability of the reflex response. Other conditions included neuronal intestinal dysplasia, aplasia of the thyroid, sigmoidal stenosis after necrotizing enterocolitis, lower rectal stenosis after perforation of rectum, sacral meningocele, and severe chronic enterocolitis.

Rectoanal Reflex in Postoperative Cases. Only three of the 21 patients with Hirschsprung's disease on whom Swenson's procedure was used demonstrated the ordinary reflex response, and in each of these, at the time of examination, over 5 years

Table 1. Rectoanal reflex in postoperative cases

	Anal canal relaxation			
	Positive	%	<10 cm H_2O	%
Hirschsprung's disease				
Swenson's procedure	3/ 21	14	–	
Soave-Denda procedure	32/ 82	39	–	
Total	35/103			
Imperforate anus				
Low type				
Primary perineal anoplasty	29/ 29	100	4/29	14
Secondary perineal anoplasty	7/ 7	100	2/ 7	29
High type				
Abdominoperineal approach	2/ 10		2/10	
Rehbein's procedure	4/ 10		3/10	
Abdominal-extended sacroperineal approach[a]	3/ 5		3/ 5	
Total	45/ 61		14/61	

[a] The reflex was measured 5 years postoperatively
Reoperative cases in low type and most cases in high type showed slight relaxation of anal canal under 10 cm H_2O

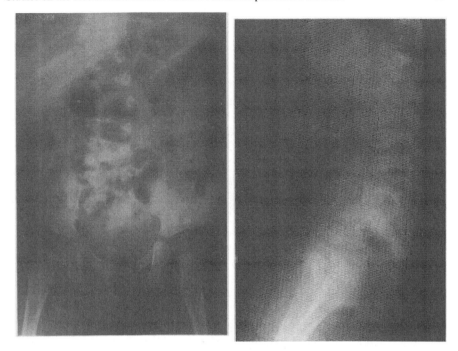

Fig. 4. The patient displays a wedge-shaped vertebra and severe sacral dysplasia

had elapsed since the operation. On the other hand, 32 cases out of 82 (39%) treated using the Soave-Denda procedure showed the reflex response from early periods after the operation (Table 1). In cases of imperforate anus, the examination indicated a prompt reflex response in all low-type cases after perineal anoplasty. Of the reoperative cases after an inappropriate initial operation, however, 29% showed only slight relaxation of anal-canal pressure, under 10 cm H_2O. While high-type anomalies did not show invariable response by the rectal stimulation, the results seemed to be more dependent on the different operative procedures. In 25 cases of high-type anomalies in which we could examine the rectoanal reflex, nine demonstrated a reflex response, although the responses almost never showed the typical pattern. With regard to the operative procedure used in these cases, a reflex was observed in two cases out of ten classical abdominoperineal operations, four cases out of ten with the Rehbein procedure, and three cases out of five with our original abdomino-extended sacroperineal approach (Yokoyama and Katsumata 1985). One case without a reflex after the Rehbein procedure had urinal incontinence preoperatively and a severe congenital sacral dysplasia (Fig. 4). The patient showed markedly low anal-canal pressure at rest postoperatively, so it is likely that this hypotonicity of the anal canal prevented a correct response from being recorded.

From all of above clinical evidence, two conditions which are necessary for appearance of the rectoanal reflex are normal intramural ganglion cells and an intact pelvic plexus. In the operative procedures which preserve the pelvic plexus, i.e., those of Soave-Denda and Rehbein and our original abdomino-extended sacroperineal approach, the incidence of rectoanal reflex was much higher than that in the simple pull-through procedure, which may cause denervation of the pelvic plexus. A third condition is that the anal-canal pressure at rest must be maintained at a normal level. None of the cases with low anal-canal pressure, as observed in sepsis and in sacral dysplasia, showed a prompt reflex response.

The reason for the high incidence of reflex response in cases with preserved pelvic plexus we must consider to be the neural mechanism of the inhibitory response in the anal canal induced by rectal distension, whether it is solely an enteric reflex mediated exclusively by intramural ganglion cells, or whether it also depends somehow upon spinal networks. Therefore, the experimental studies described in the next section were carried out to define the precise factors eliciting the reflex response.

Experimental Studies

Material and Methods

Experiments were done on 36 dogs, each weighing about 10 kg. Of these, 27 were used for short-term studies and 9 for long-term observation of sacral denervation. For animals in the short-term experimental group, decerebration was carried out at the midcollicular level under thiopental sodium anesthesia (20 mg/kg, intravenously). After manometric measurement of the ordinary rectoanal reflex, the spinal cord was exposed at the lumbosacral level. The electrical activities of the internal and external anal sphincters were recorded continuously by stainless-steel bipolar electrodes inserted into each muscle as a floating electrode, and the intraluminal pressure within the anal canal was simultaneously recorded with our original probe. The exposed sacral roots, from the first to the third, were stimulated through bipolar platinum electrodes with repetitive electric pulses, either extradurally or intradurally, instead of being stimulated with the rectal balloon. The nine dogs in the long-term study were anesthetized deeply with an intravenous injection of phentobarbital sodium (Nembutal; 40 mg/kg) on the 1st day of the experiment, and their exposed sacral roots, from the first to the third, were sectioned bilaterally through an extradural approach. Thereafter, most of the dogs were kept alive over 1 month with careful follow-up of their defecatory behaviour. On the final experimental day, they were decerebrated under short-acting anesthesia of thiopental sodium (15 mg/kg intravenous) in order to compare their reflex responses with those obtained in sacral-intact dogs.

Results of Experimental Studies

Correlation Between Electrical Activity of the Internal Sphincter and the Rectoanal Reflex. When a transient drop in anal-canal pressure was induced by rectal disten-

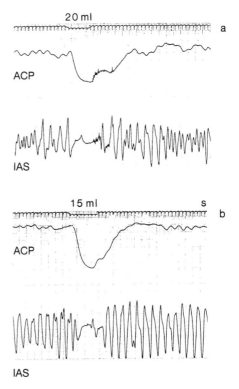

Fig. 5a, b. Responses of rectal distension in a dog before (**a**) and after (**b**) the injection of 2 mg/kg somatic neuromuscular blocking agent succinylcholine chloride. The injection did not cause any alteration in pressure levels or internal sphincter slow-spike rate (**b**). *ACP*, anal canal pressure; *IAS*, internal and sphincter spikes

sion, the so-called rhythmical waves in pressure, which we call "ripples," and the slow spikes due to the internal sphincters disappeared at once and then reappeared simultaneously in manometric and myoelectrical recordings during the recovery phase of the reflex (Fig. 5). Intravenous injection of the "somatic" neuro-muscular blocking agent succinylcholine chloride did not essentially change the pattern of responses (Fig. 5b).

The graded increase in distension volume induced in the rectum brought about progressive lengthening of the time during which the internal sphincter spikes were inhibited, causing prolongation of the falling phase of pressure in the rectoanal reflex (Fig. 6). The same phenomena were seen when giving electrical stimulation to the distal cut end of the second sacral ventral root. The inhibition of internal sphincter spikes, elicited by electrical stimulation, was prolonged gradationally in parallel with the increase in stimulus strength. Inhibition of the internal sphincter lasted for 5s by stimulation with 0.3 V and for 10s with 0.4 V (Fig. 7). Furthermore, simultaneous application of rectal distension via the balloon and electric pulses to the first ventral root of sacral nerve brought about a complete inhibition of sustained slow spikes and a rapid fall in anal-canal pressure, with disappearance of pressure ripples, as shown in Fig. 8. This observation indicates a summation of stimulations delivered simultaneously by different modes and from different places.

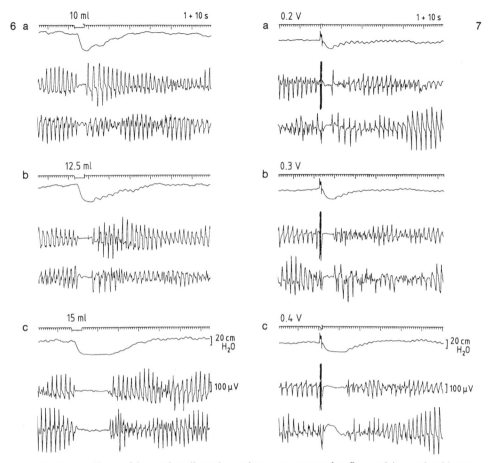

Fig. 6a–c. Effects of increasing distension volume on rectoanal reflex and internal sphincter spikes. A constant distension time of 5 s was used, and a distension volume of 10 ml (**a**), 12.5 ml (**b**), and 15 ml (**c**) was employed in the rectum, using a thiopental sodium anesthetized, decerebrated dog. *Uppermost lines* of each trace indicate the time mark in each recording

Fig. 7a–c. Effects of increasing strength of electrical stimulation of the distal cut end of the second sacral ventral root on internal sphincter spikes. **a** 0.2 V. **b** 0.3 V. **c** 0.4 V. Stimulating pulses were 0.1 ms; stimulating frequency was 10 Hz, and time interval was 1 s. The dog (7.5 kg) was anesthetized with thiopental sodium

Quantitative Differences in Rectoanal Response to Distension in Sacrally Denervated Dogs. As shown in Fig. 9a, the rectoanal reflex was obtained promptly from sacral-intact decerebrate dogs. The tracing of anal-canal pressure exhibited successive ripples, the rate of which was consistent with slow-spike potentials recorded from internal anal sphincters. Following the rectal distension with 10 ml air, the sustained slow spikes and the pressure ripples were inhibited completely, accompanied by a rapid fall in anal-canal pressure. After a 10-s fall in pressure and in-

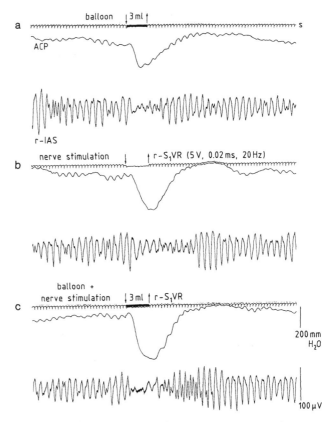

Fig. 8. a Reflex response to rectal distension by 3 ml air. **b** Reaction upon electric pulses (5 V, 0.02 ms, 20 Hz) to the first ventral root of sacral nerve *(r-S_1VR)*. **c** Reflex response combining the two modes of stimulation. *ACP*, Anal canal pressure; *r-IAS*, right internal anal sphincter spikes

hibition of slow spikes of internal sphincters, the ripples and slow spikes reappeared consistently, regaining their former rhythmus rapidly.

In a dog decerebrated on the 42nd day after sacral denervation, the rate of slow spikes decreased, and the pressure ripples became larger in size during resting activity. The altered behavior of the anal canal after sacral denervation was more distinct in the elicited rectoanal reflex: prolonged inhibition of slow spikes, retarded course of recovery, and marked formation of rebound were seen in response to the rectal distension (Fig. 9b).

Furthermore, the response of the anal canal to graded extents of rectal distension were compared in detail in "intact" dogs and in "denervated" dogs. The records of Fig. 10a–c were obtained from "intact" dogs and the records d–f from "denervated" dogs decerebrated on the 28th day after nerve sectioning. The differences in resting activity between intact and denervated dogs are again evident. The spike rate in the former was about 30 per second in contrast to about 20 per

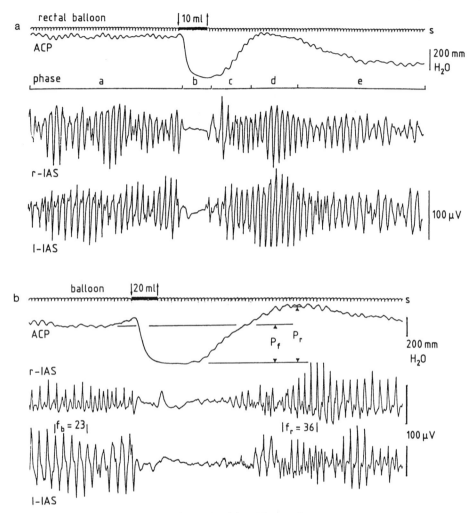

Fig. 9a, b. The reflex response in intact dog (**a**) and in sacrally denervated (**b**) dog (42 days after S_{1-13} denervation). *ACP,* Anal canal pressure; *r-IAS* and *l-IAS,* right and left internal anal sphincter spikes, respectively

second in the latter; these rates reflected the corresponding rates and, inversely, the size of pressure ripples. The gradational nature of reflex responses to threshold stimuli (a and d), to suprathreshold stimuli (b and e), and to near-maximal stimuli (c and f) was more apparent in intact dogs than in denervated dogs, being indicated by the duration of slow-spike inhibition. This duration of inhibition was independent of the duration of rectal distension but increased in proportion to the distension volume in "intact" dogs (b and c). By contrast, in "denervated" dogs it increased abruptly up to 17 s with a distension of 15 ml (e), and an additional 5 ml distension brought about an inhibition of 22 s (f). Such prolonged inhibition has scarcely been attained in "intact" dogs even by the maximal volume of distension.

Discussion

Our findings demonstrate that rectoanal reflex is not recognized in cases with aganglionic bowel and in postoperative cases in which pelvic nerve plexuses may be damaged. However, when patients are not physiologically normal, as in sepsis or hypothyroidism, the rectoanal reflex is affected. Therefore, the decision as to whether the rectoanal reflex is present or not should be made only after examination of the patient under normal physiological conditions.

If the neural pathway of rectoanal reflex is mediated only by intramural ganglion cells, in all of the postoperative rectoanal deformities and Hirschsprung's disease, the anal canal pressure should show the relaxation by rectal distension because the normal colon is pulled through in both operative methods. However, the clinical results as described above can only be explained by the additional regulation by the sacral pathway.

Bouvier and Gonella (1981a, b) demonstrated that in humans the slow potentials of internal sphincters disappeared, accompanied by a fall in anal-canal pressure. However, their studies did not clearly define the correlation between anal-canal pressure and the "slow spike" potentials of internal sphincters because the effects of anesthesia influenced the slow spikes and pressures in the anal canal; in the clinical setting, it is very difficult to show clearly the correlation between anal-canal pressure and electrical activity of the internal sphincter. Therefore, we performed studies using dogs decerebrated at the midcollicular level.

When a transient drop in anal-canal pressure was induced by rectal distension, slow spikes of internal sphincters disappeared at once and reappeared simultaneously during the recovery phase of the reflex, as seen from the manometric recordings. It is concluded, therefore, that the slow spikes of the internal sphincters are directly coupled with the mechanical response of these muscles, that the sustained contraction of internal sphincters maintains the pressure level of the anal canal, and that their temporary relaxation causes the pressure to fall. Further, intravenous injection of a somatic neuromuscular blocking agent did not cause any alteration in pressure level and slow spike rate of the internal sphincters. This evidence indicates that anal-canal pressure is primarily dependent on sustained activity of internal sphincters, not on tonic discharge of external sphincters.

The phenomena elicited by electrical stimulation of the sacral nerve were identified as constituting the same response as the rectoanal reflex by rectal distension, and the two different simultaneous stimulations, mechanical and electrical, showed effects of summation by bringing about a complete inhibition of slow spikes of internal sphincters. This indicates that neuronal impulses from the sacral network bring about complete inhibition of internal sphincter activity via myenteric inhibitory neurons.

The studies presented by Gowers (1877) and Denny-Brown and Robertson (1935) were designed to seek clues to the mechanism of the rectoanal reflex, specifi-

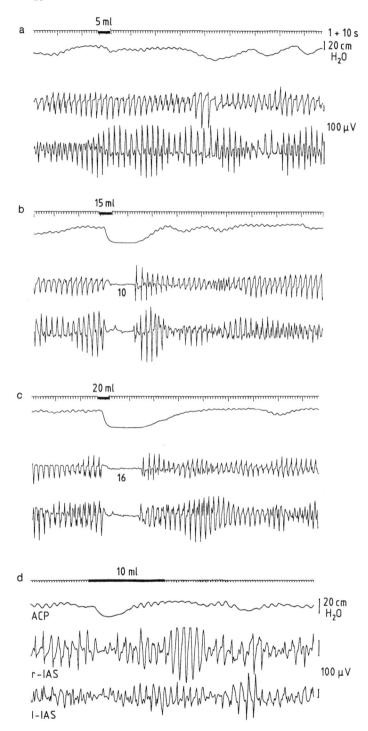

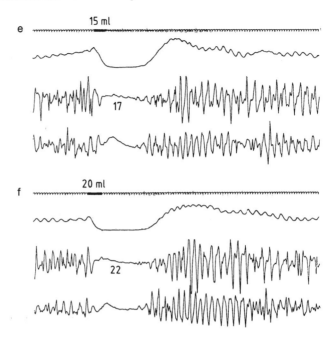

Fig. 10a–f. Rectoanal reflexes in response to graded increases in rectal distension. **a–c** Records from intact dogs. **d–f** Records from denervated dogs. Volume and duration of rectal distension are indicated on the upper most line of the time mark in each record. Numbers below the *r-IAS* traces in **b, c, e,** and **f** indicate the duration of complete inhibition (in seconds)

cally whether the reflex depends on only myenteric plexuses. However, they could not clearly demonstrate any correlation between the myenteric plexuses and the sacral nerves because only clinical materials were used in their studies; in these clinical cases of spinal trauma it thus could not be decided clearly which level of the spine was impaired. Therefore, if we discuss the hypothesis in light of clinical data only, we can not obtain any definite conclusion.

The most remarkable features of anal-canal activity resulting from sacral denervation were (a) prolonged inhibition of slow spikes in the rectoanal reflex and marked formation of reflex rebound and (b) the decreasing rate of rhythmical waves of the anal canal corresponding to the decreasing rate of slow spikes of internal sphincters. It is likely that the lower rate of resting activity of slow spikes (Figs. 9b, 10) may induce the altered behavior of the anal canal in denervated dogs. It is further suggested that the myenteric inhibitory neurons are potentiated when they are isolated from the sacral innervation.

Meunier and Mollard (1976, 1977) demonstrated low resting pressure of the anal canal in cases with myelomeningocele. Furthermore, this case showed the characteristics of the reflex response similar to those seen with our sacrally denervated dogs.

From the results of our clinical and experimental studies, we have schematized the neuronal pathway of the rectoanal reflex, as shown in Fig. 11. In a normally

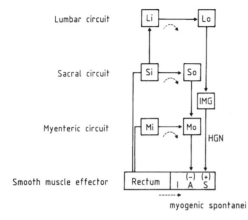

Fig. 11. Proposed diagram of the neuronal pathway of rectoanal reflex. (Concerning the lumbar circuit, we have shown no data in this report relating to its involvement). *Li, Si, Mi,* input neurons; *Lo, So, Mo,* output neurons; *IMG,* hypogastric ganglia; *HGN,* hypogastric nerves; *(−)* inhibitory action; *(+),* acceleratory action

innervated condition, the stimulation by rectal distension induces a transient drop in pressure in the anal canal via the sacral cord and myenteric neurons. In other words, the normal rectoanal reflex is mediated by both the sacral cord and the myenteric neurons. Therefore, we think that measurements of the resting pressure of the anal canal and the rectoanal reflex constitute a very valuable method to decide whether the patient has normal sacral and myenteric innervation.

References

Boley SJ, Lafer DJ, Klenhaus S (1968) Endorectal pull-through procedure for Hirschsprung's disease with and without primary anastomosis. J Pediatr Surg 3:258–262

Bouvier M, Gonella J (1981a) Electrical activity from smooth muscle of the anal sphincteric area of the cat. J Physiol (Lond) 310:445–456

Bouvier M, Gonella J (1981b) Nervous control of the internal anal sphincter of the cat. J Physiol (Lond) 310:457–469

Denda T (1965) The therapy of Hirschsprung's disease. J Keio Med Soc 42:379–388

Denny-Brown D, Robertson EG (1935) An investigation of the nervous control of defecation. Brain 58:256–310

Gaston EA (1948) The physiology of fecal continence. Surg Gynecol Obstet 87:280–290

Gowers WR (1877) The automatic action of the sphincter ani. Proc R Soc Lond 26:77–84

Holschneider AM (1974) Elektromyographische Untersuchungen der Musculi sphincter ani externus und internus im Bezug auf die anorektale Manometrie. Langenbecks Arch Chir 333:303–316

Ikeda K (1966) New techniques for Hirschsprung's disease. J Jpn Soc Pediatr Surg 2:38–39

Ito Y, Yokoyama J (1981) Reappraisal of endorectal pull-through procedure I. J Pediatr Surg 16:476–483

Lawson JON, Nixon HH (1967) Anal canal pressure in the diagnosis of Hirschsprung's disease. J Pediatr Surg 2:544–552

Meunier P, Mollard P (1976) Manometric studies of anorectal disorders in infancy and childhood: an investigation of the physiopathology of continence and defecation. Br J Surg 63:402–407

Meunier P, Mollard P (1977) Control of the internal anal sphincter: manometric study with human subjects. Pflügers Arch 370:233–239

Nixon HH (1978) Operative surgery, pediatric surgery, 3rd edn. Butterworths, London, p 135

Schnaufer L, Talbert JL (1967) Differential sphincteric studies in the diagnosis of anorectal disorders of childhood. J Pediatr Surg 2:538–543

Yokoyama J, Katsumata K (1985) Abdomino-extended sacroperineal approach in high type anorectal malformation − and a new operative method. Z Kinderchir 40:151–157

Computerized Analysis of Anorectal Manometry

M. Sakaniwa, S. Sawaguchi, H. Ohkawa, and K. Ikebukuro

Summary

A computer system was designed and applied to anorectal manometry that allows pressure data to be analysed in various ways. Two kinds of applications were presented. Image analysis enabled anorectal movements to be visualized as a three-dimensional image. This technique was shown to be useful in studying the pathophysiology of chronic constipation in children. Radial variation analysis demonstrated that there was no significant radial difference in the anal-canal pressure.

Zusammenfassung

Es wurde ein Computersystem für die anorektale Manometrie entwickelt, das verschiedene Analysen der Manometriedaten ermöglicht. Zwei Anwendungsgebiete werden beschrieben. Die Bildanalyse erlaubt die dreidimensionale Darstellung der anorektalen Bewegungsabläufe und erweist sich somit als wertvolle Technik zum Studium der Pathophysiologie der chronischen Obstipation im Kindesalter. Die Druckvektoranalyse ergab keine signifikanten Unterschiede der Druckvektoren im Analkanal.

Résumé

Une informatisation de la manométrie anorectale a été mise au point, permettant ainsi une analyse multicentrique des résultats de la manométrie. Les auteurs décrivent deux champs d'application. L'analyse des images permet une représentation tridimensionnelle des mouvements anorectaux, apportant une aide précieuse dans l'étude des aspects physiopathologiques de la constipation chronique de l'enfant. L'analyse de la variation des vecteurs de pression n'a pas montré de différence significative entre ceux du canal anal.

It has been well recognized that anorectal manometry is a useful tool not only for diagnosing Hirschsprung's disease but also for investigating the motility of the anorectum. Conditions for studying exact pressure changes have been meticulously investigated (Maie et al. 1978), and many sophisticated modifications in both the catheters and the pressure-recording systems (Arndorfer et al. 1977) have been introduced in order to obtain more detailed information. We have designed and applied a computer system to anorectal manometry that allows all the data to

Department of Paediatric Surgery, Institute of Clinical Medicine, University of Tsukuba, 1-1-1 Amakubo, Sakura-mura, Niihari-gun, Ibaraki-ken 305, Japan

be stored digitally in a computer memory. This system has enabled us to make a variety of analyses using the data collected.

Materials and Methods

Pressure-Recording System

Two types of pressure probes were newly designed. The first was a longitudinal probe, composed of four polyethylene tubes (Fig. 1, A: a, b, c and d; inner diameter 1 mm; single laterally placed openings) bonded on a rubber tube (outer diameters 4.2 mm) with distal side openings 0.5 cm apart. This probe was inserted into the anus with the side holes facing posteriorly and placed so that pressures at 2, 1.5, 1.0 and 0.5 cm from the anal margin could be measured simultaneously. The second was a cross-sectional probe, a four-lumen catheter used to measure cross-sectional pressure changes in the anal canal (Fig. 1, B). This probe was placed with side openings facing the anterior, posterior, right and left side of the anal canal. The openings were positioned in the upper anal canal where the rhythmical activities of the anal canal were best recorded. The size and material of the tubes were the same in both probe types. Each channel was connected to a pneumohydraulic infusion system (Arndorfer et al. 1977). Four pairs of pressure transducers (HP-1290A) and amplifiers (HP-78801A) were used. The fifth tube, (Fig. 1, e), with a rubber balloon at the tip, was inserted through the lumen of the rubber tube. The balloon was inflated with air to stimulate the rectal wall in order to induce the rectoanal inhibitory (RAI) reflex. Balloon distension was maintained for at least 5 s. The initial amount of air ranged from 3 ml in neonates and infants to 5 ml in older patients. The amounts were gradually increased. If the RAI reflex was shown to be positive, the amount of air was increased until no larger relaxation was observed. The relaxation index of the RAI reflex was calculated by dividing the pressure difference between the anal-canal pressure immediately before the rectal distension (Pr) and the lowest point of the relaxation by the

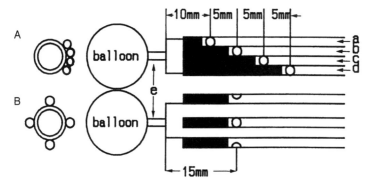

Fig. 1. Longitudinal *(A)* cross-sectional *(B)* probes

anal-canal pressure determined as Pr. The largest value obtained was termed the maximal relaxation index.

Computer System

The outputs of the four pressure amplifiers were fed into an analog-to-digital converter (ADM-1008 Adtech Science, Japan). The data were sampled once every second, converted into 8-digit number within 2.2 µs and fed into a microcomputer (Apple-II or NEC PC-9801U2). When the longitudinal probe was used, the pressure profiles of the anal canal were displayed on a cathode ray tube on a real-time basis. After the examination, all the data obtained were stored on a floppy disc. Subsequently, analyses were made by the computer using these data. Pictures of the image produced were printed by either a graphic printer (MP-80 Epson) or a X-Y plotter (DXY-980 Roland DG, Japan).

Clinical Materials

The examination was performed on 27 patients with chronic constipation, 15 patients with Hirschsprung's disease and another 20 patients with miscellaneous disorders, including anorectal malformations, myelomeningocele and colon polyp. Ages ranged between 11 days and 12 years. The average age was 3 years and 4 months ± 37 months (mean ± SD). There were 34 boys and 28 girls. In patients with Hirschsprung's disease, preoperative examinations were carried out seven times on five patients, and postoperative examinations were performed ten times on six patients who had had the modified Soave's operation (Boley's procedure), once on a patient after the original Soave's operation, and five times on three patients who had had the modified Duhamel's operation (Martin's procedure, two cases; Ikeda's procedure, one case). All of the patients were orally sedated with monosodium trichlorethyl phosphate, 100 mg/kg, with an upper limit of 1 g. Patients were placed on their right side. Image analyses were made on all the patients, whereas radial variation analyses were made on only seven patients with chronic constipation and one postoperative patient with Hirschsprung's disease who had had the modified Soave's operation (Boley's procedure).

Computerized Analyses

Image Analysis (Dynamic Pressure Profile Imaging). Pressure profiles of the anal canal were plotted at 1-s intervals using pressure values of 2, 1.5, 1 and 0.5 cm from the anal margin and were arranged on the time axis. They formed a three-dimensional image as shown in Fig. 2. In this image, time was shown on the horizontal axis (A), distance from the anal margin on the lateral axis (B), and the pressure value on the vertical axis (C). By appropriately modifying the computer programme, the same data was illustrated in several forms (Fig. 3, A, B and C).

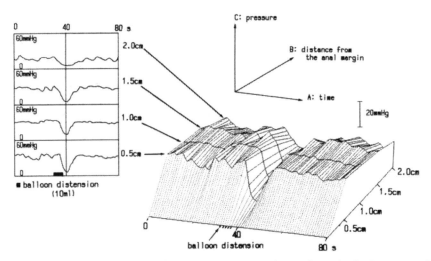

Fig. 2. Three-dimensional image processing. Pressure change shown in the linear recording on the left is displayed as a three-dimensional image on the right. (Normal control, 3-year-old girl)

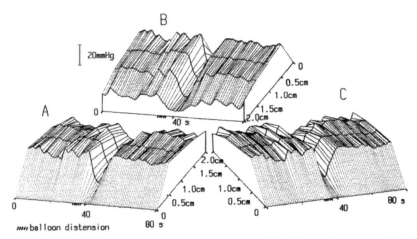

Fig. 3. Images seen from different points of view. Note that *B* is a mirror image of *A*. (Normal control same as in Fig. 2)

In this way, it was possible to study points of particular interest in detail. This technique is referred to here as dynamic pressure profile imaging.

Radial Variation Analysis (Pressure Vector Analysis). Cross-sectional pressure values for 40 s were plotted on the X-Y ordinates. Four points for each second were connected with the spline curve. To demonstrate the direction and the value of the radial pressure difference, the pressure vector was calculated and plotted

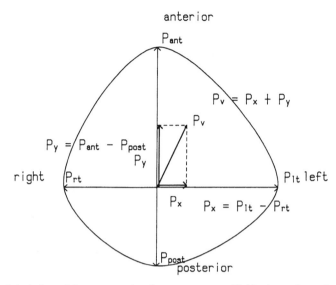

Fig. 4. Calculation of the cross-sectional pressure vector *(Pv)* in the anal canal

on the X-Y axis. This vector was the sum of the following two vectors: the rightward vector, which was the difference between the right pressure and the left pressure, and the upward vector, which was the difference between the anterior pressure and posterior pressure (Fig. 4). If there was no radial variation in the anal-canal pressure, this vector was to be nil.

Results

Reproducibility of the Rectoanal Inhibitory Reflex

To investigate how reproducible the pressure profiles from one rectal stimulation to another were, the amount of air used to distend the balloon in the rectum was changed at several steps in all of the constipated patients. No patient showed any significant variations in the shape of the RAI reflex, and neither did their dynamic pressure profile images show any significant variations. As more air was placed in the balloon in the rectum, there was an apparent tendency for the RAI reflex to increase. However, the depth of the relaxations induced was not strictly proportional to the amount of air (Fig. 5).

Image Analysis

Chronic Constipation

The visualized images of the RAI reflex in the constipated children were generally classified into three types according to the following two points: the amplitude of

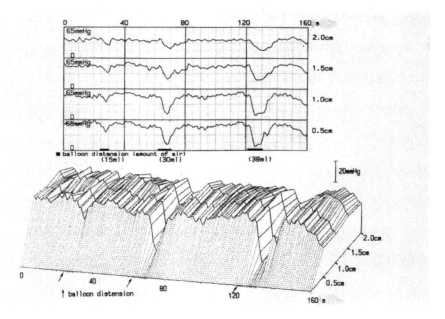

Fig. 5. Reproducibility of the RAI reflex. As the amount of air used to distend the balloon was increased from 15 ml to 38 ml, the RAI reflex became larger and larger, maintaining a similar shape. (Chronic constipation, 3-year-old boy)

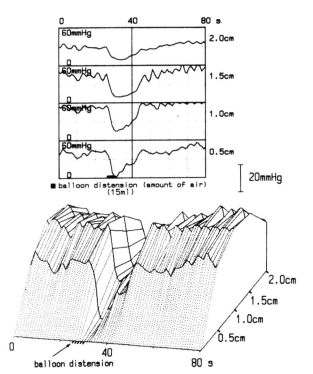

Fig. 6. Chronic constipation, type 1. (3-year-old boy)

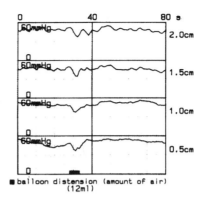

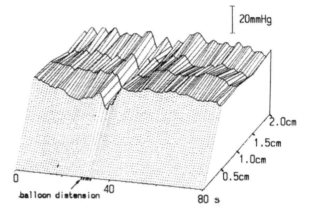

Fig. 7. Chronic constipation, type 2. (3-year-old boy)

the rhythmical activities in the anal canal, and the shape and depth of the relaxations during the reflex. The type 1 image was similar to those of normal children (Fig. 6; cf. Figs. 2, 3 for normal image). There were 14 patients included in this group. The maximal relaxation index was 0.80 ± 0.01 (mean ± SD). The type 2 image was of those in which the depth of the relaxations were significantly small even in the maximal relaxations. This type of image was seen in 14 patients. These cases were more clearly demonstrated in the dynamic pressure profile image than in the linear chart. The RAI reflex was shown as a shallow notch in these images (Fig. 7). The maximal relaxation index was 0.53 ± 0.01 (mean ± SD) and significantly smaller than in the type 1 group ($P < 0.01$). The type 3 image was of those in which the amplitude of the rhythmical activities were significantly large (Fig. 8). Three patients showed this type of image. The maximal relaxation index ranged from 0.71 to 1.0.

There were three patients who underwent repeated examinations while receiving treatment for constipation on an outpatient basis. Two patients showed changes in the image type during the clinical course of treatment. An 8-year-old boy showed type 3 on the first examination and then type 1 2 months later while having bowel movements by enema. On the third examination 2 months later when he began to soil his underwear, he showed type 2 image. A 3-year-old boy showed type 1 on

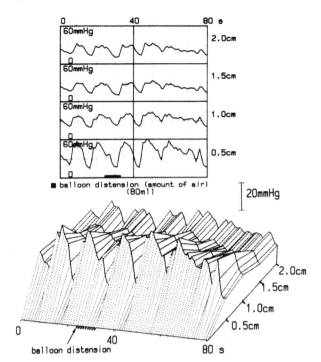

Fig. 8. Chronic constipation, type 3. (10-year-old boy)

the first examination, type 2 2 weeks later, and then type 1 2 years and 7 months later. He had had almost regular bowel movements by laxatives and enemas until he began to soil himself a year later. The image that was produced upon examination, however, remained in the type 1 category.

Hirschsprung's Disease

Preoperative Results. Four patients had examinations during infancy. In these patients, repeated rectal distension did not produce any remarkable changes in any of the rhythmical activities 0.5–2.0 cm from the anal margin. A boy, aged 3 years, who had had severe constipation from birth showed abnormal rhythmical activities. The wave was significantly large in size, and its frequency was as slow as 6.0 cycles per minute. (The normal value is 13.5 ± 3.9 cycle per minute in the upper anal canal; Sakaniwa et al. 1979). Upon rectal stimulation, there was a small decrease in pressure in the distal anal canal. However, the dynamic pressure profile imaging of this recording demonstrated that the anal canal as a whole did not relax well enough (Fig. 9). This pressure decrease was differentiated from both that of a normal response image and the constipation type 2 image. Rectal biopsy revealed the aganglionosis.

Postoperative Results. The examination was performed on 10 patients. The RAI reflex was absent in all cases. One patient, who had had a modified Soave's opera-

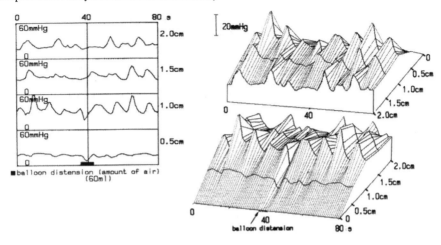

Fig. 9. Hirschsprung's disease, before operation. (3-year-old boy)

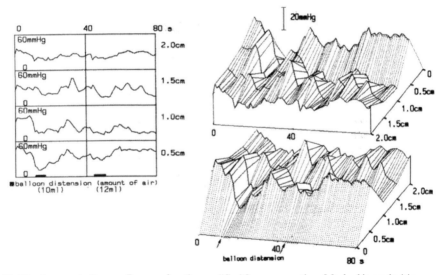

Fig. 10. Hirschsprung's disease, 7 years after the modified Soave operation. Marked irregularities in the waves are seen in the middle and upper anal canal. (Boy, 7 years and 7 months old)

tion 7 years prior to the examination, began to soil himself and was referred for the examination. In dynamic imaging, the rhythmical activities looked almost regular in the distal anal canal. But these rhythmical activities in the middle and the upper anal canal seemed to be working irregularly without any coordination. There was a pressure gap between the distal portion and the rest of the anal canal (Fig. 10).

Radial Variation Analysis (Pressure Vector Analysis)

The circle-like images made by combining the four pressure values maintained similar shapes during both the resting state and the RAI reflex. In all patients except two examined with constipation, the images were almost symmetric in the four directions. The pressure vectors were very small in size, and their directions remained with in a narrow range (Fig. 11a). In two patients who showed slight

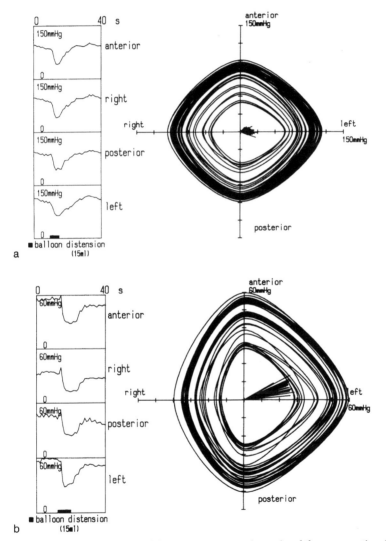

Fig. 11a, b. Multiplotting of the pressure vectors *(centre)* and the cross-sectional pressure profiles *(oval curves)* for 40 s. **a** Chronic constipation, 10-year-old boy. **b** Chronic constipation, 6-year-old boy

asymmetry, the left-anterior pressure was more dominant (Fig. 11b). In a postoperative case of Hirschsprung's disease the image was symmetric.

Discussion

The dynamic pressure profile imaging described here enabled the anorectal activities to be visualized in three-dimensional pictures. These pictures give a good understanding of anorectal motilities. Theoretically, the linear chart recording contains comprehensive information which an examination may obtain. But it takes a good deal of work and an experienced eye to acknowledge what meaning the chart recording holds. The displayed image is far easier to understand even for a beginner once he is informed how to read it. One of the disadvantages of this imaging may be that it is not possible to measure the actual pressure from the image. But this imaging is not meant to substitute totally for the conventional recordings. The important point is that this imaging can offer new kinds of information which conventional chart reading cannot disclose.

In this study, manometric analysis was made on chronic constipation in children. It should be emphasized that the whole population of those experiencing chronic constipation is not homogeneous in regards to pathology (Martelli et al. 1978; Arhan et al. 1983; Frieri et al. 1983; Shouler and Keighley 1986; Ducrotte et al. 1986; Meunier 1986). This imaging enabled us to differentiate those patients with internal anal sphincter abnormalities. Although there was no remarkable feature in the type 1 image compared with the normal control, the type 2 image showed poor relaxation of the anal canal. This indicates that relaxation of the internal anal sphincter in these patients is unsatisfactory. Loening-Baucke (1984) reported that, statistically, the percent relaxation of the RAI reflex was lower in constipated children than in control cases. Our results partly confirm this. Although we have no experience in the surgical treatment of idiopathic chronic constipation thus far, we consider those patients who show this type of image to be possible candidates for surgery such as internal sphincterectomy. The type 3 group also indicated abnormal internal anal sphincter motilities, as the rhythmical activities represented basal activity of the internal anal sphincter (Wankling et al. 1968; Ihara and Takahira 1984). However, relaxation of the internal anal sphincter was normal, judging from the maximal relaxation index. Clear explanation for this large amplitude of the internal anal sphincter activity retaining good relaxation ability in the RAI reflex is unknown at the present time. We have seen similar patterns in the rhythmical activities in patients with myelomeningocele (Sakaniwa et al. 1981). Although these patients classified as type 3 here were not found to have had apparent neurological disturbances, there was a possibility that some unrevealed local neurological factor(s) played a role in their diseases.

Suzuki et al. (1981) showed there was no significant radial difference in the anorectal pressure. Taylor et al. (1984), on the contrary, reported that the anal canal had marked, but consistent, radial and longitudinal variations in pressure. Our results of the pressure vector analysis demonstrated that there was no such radial variation. This is quite consistent with the principle of physics. According to Pascal's law, pressure in a closed space is uniform. If the radial pressure difference is detected at any point in the anal canal, it should be made by distortion by some artifact, for example, the force produced by the rigidity of the catheter, which is unevenly attached to the anal canal. If a pressure vector should exist, the catheter should move in the vector's direction. The reason why it does not move is that there is another force working from the reverse direction.

Here we have presented two kinds of computerized analyses of anorectal manometry. We would like to emphasize that this computerized manometric system is very useful, and that many applications of this system are feasible in investigating anorectal motilities.

Acknowledgement. The authors are grateful to Miss L. Bond for her kind help in preparing the manuscript.

References

Arhan P, Devroede G, Jehannin B, Faverdin C, Revillon Y, Lefevre D, Pellerin D (1983) Idiopathic disorders of fecal continence in children. Pediatrics 71:774–779

Arndorfer RC, Stol JJ, Dodds WJ, Linehan JH, Hogan WJ (1977) Improved infusion system for intraluminal esophageal manometry. Gastroenterology 73:23–27

Ducrotte P, Rodomanska B, Weber J, Guillard JF, Lerebours E, Hecketsweiler P, Galmiche JP, Colin R, Denis P (1986) Colonic transit time of radiopaque markers and rectoanal manometry in patients complaining of constipation. Dis Colon Rectum 29:630–634

Frieri G, Parisi F, Corazziari E, Caprlli R (1983) Colonic electromyography in chronic constipation. Gastroenterology 84:737–740

Ihara N, Takahira H (1984) Regulation of anal canal pressure as revealed by myoelectrical activity of internal anal sphincter. Jpn J Smooth Muscle Res 20:123–135

Loening-Baucke VA (1984) Abnormal rectoanal function in children recovered from chronic constipation and encopresis. Gastroenterology 87:1299–1304

Maie M, Iino M, Sakaniwa M, Ohkawa H, Takahashi H (1978) Conditions for studying the exact pressure changes in the alimentary tract. Prog Pediatr Surg 12:165–183

Martelli H, Devroede G, Arhan P, Duguay C (1978) Mechanisms of idiopathic constipation: outlet obstruction. Gastroenterology 75:623–631

Meunier P (1986) Physiologic study of the terminal digestive tract in chronic painful constipation. Gut 27:1018–1024

Sakaniwa M, Takahashi H, Maie M, Ohnuma N, Nakajima K, Ihno M, Aoyagi H, Iwai J (1979) Ano-rectal manometry with an infused open-tip method – the first report, the standard values of normal cases. J Jpn Soc Colon Rectum 32:324–335

Sakaniwa M, Takahashi H, Maie M, Ohkawa H, Yamane Y (1981) Manometric studies on the anorectal function in myelomeningocele. J Jpn Soc Pediatr Surg 17:635–642

Shouler P, Keighley MRB (1986) Changes in colorectal function in severe idiopathic chronic constipation. Gastroenterology 90:414–420

Suzuki H, Honzumi M, Amano S, Kuroda M (1981) Contribution to anorectal manometry with side-opening catheter. Z Kinderchir 34:87–89

Taylor BM, Beart RW, Phillips SF (1984) Longitudinal and radial variations of pressure in the human anal sphincter. Gastroenterology 86:693–697

Wankling WJ, Brown BH, Collins CD, Duthie HL (1968) Basal electrical activity in the anal canal in man. Gut 9:457–460

The Electromyographic Examination to Evaluate the External Sphincter Muscle in Anorectal Malformations

A. Hayashi[1], J. Yokoyama[2], and K. Katsumata[2]

Summary

Preoperative electromyographic examination is very useful in locating the external sphincter muscles and determining their degree of development. Electromyographic examinations showed the relatively abundant distribution of the external sphincter muscles in the perineum even in high-type anomalies. The results obtained by these examinations lead to the conclusion that preserving both the puborectal and external sphincter muscles should be the main consideration in surgery for anorectal malformations.

Zusammenfassung

Die präoperative Elektromyographie ist eine sehr nützliche Methode zur Lokalisation des externen Sphinkterapparates und zur Bestimmung seines Entwicklungsgrades. Elektromyographische Untersuchungen ergaben ein relativ häufiges Vorhandensein des externen Sphinkters im Dammbereich – sogar bei den hohen Formen der anorektalen Fehlbildungen. Die Ergebnisse aus diesen Untersuchungen führen zu dem Schluß, daß die Erhaltung sowohl des M. puborectalis als auch des externen Sphinkters das Hauptziel bei Operationen an anorektalen Fehlbildungen sein muß.

Résumé

L'électromyographie préopératoire est une méthode de choix pour localiser les muscles du sphincter externe et déterminer leur degré de développement. Les examens électromyographiques ont montré la présence relativement fréquente du sphincter externe au niveau du perinée même dans le cas de malformations anorectales très haut placées. Il ressort des résultats de ces examens que le traitement chirurgical des malformations anorectales se doit avant tout de conserver le muscle puborectal et les muscles du sphincter externe.

Introduction

The internal and external sphincters and the levator muscles govern the flow of feces and mucus in normal children. In patients with an anorectal malformation, especially those with a high-type anomaly, a normally developed internal sphincter

---

[1] Department of Surgery, Tokyo Metropolitan Kiyose Children's Hospital, 1-3-1 Umezono, Kiyose, Tokyo 204, Japan
[2] Department of Pediatric Surgery, School of Medicine, Keio University, 35 Shinanomachi, Shinjuku-Ku, Tokyo 160, Japan

muscle is absent, and only a hypertrophied internal circular muscle is present at a distal part of the rectum (Yokoyama et al. 1985). Hence, after an anorectoplasty, continence is usually ensured by the puborectal muscle, the lowest component of levator muscles, and the external sphincter muscle, even when their development is also impaired to some degree. Since Stephens and Smith (1971a) reported that the puborectal muscle played an important role in the postoperative continence of patients with an anorectal malformation, pediatric surgeons have stressed the function of this muscle in sustaining continence. However, the role of the external sphincter muscle in sustaining continence has tended to be underestimated, hampered by a basic shortage of information about this muscle in patients with anorectal malformations. This is hardly a trivial point, for it affects the surgeon's strategy during anorectoplasty. The present study provides evidence that the surgeon's chief consideration should be preserving both the puborectal and external sphincter muscles in the treatment of patients with anorectal malformations.

The location and function of external sphincter muscles in patients with anorectal malformations were determined before each operation by electromyography. Information obtained by electromyographic examination proved extremely useful for anorectoplasty operation in preserving external sphincter muscles around a newly constructed anus.

Material and Methods

The electromyographic examination was performed about 1–2 weeks before each operation. A total of 82 patients with anorectal malformations were evaluated by electromyography. Using the international classification (Santulli et al. 1970; Stephens and Smith 1971b), 50 patients were classified as having low-type anomalies, 9 as having intermediate-type, and 23 as having high-type anomalies (Table 1).

Table 1. Classification of cases in which electromyographic examinations was performed

Low-type anomalies	n	Intermediate-type anomalies	n	High-type anomalies	n
Anocutaneous	23	Anal agenesis	3	Rectourethral	12
Anovestibular	16	Rectobulbar	3	Rectovesical	5
Covered anus-complete	4	Rectovaginal (low)	2	Rectocloacal	3
Anovulvar	3	Rectovestibular	1	Anorectal agenesis	2
Covered anal-stenosis	2	Total	9	Vesicointestinal fissure	1
Unclassified	2			Total	23
Total	50				

Rectovestibular fistula is a rare type in which a long fistula between rectal pouch and vestibulum is present. Vesicointestinal fissure and rectocloacal fistula were apparently supralevator and classified as a high-type anomaly in this paper

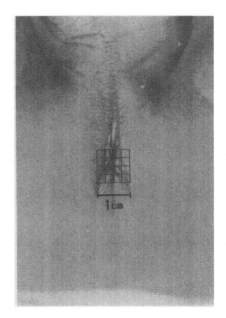

Fig. 1. The area to be examined, 1 cm². At 2.5-mm intervals 25 points, at which the needle electrode was inserted, were spaced along a grid

The average ages of patients, with low-, intermediate-, and high-type anomalies, were 6.7, 7.8, and 7.3 months, respectively.

The area to be examined was 1 cm². This was determined by the location of skin markings, specifically by either a dimple or pigmentation or both at the perineum. Within this area 25 points were spaced along a grid at 2.5-mm intervals, as shown in Fig. 1. At these points a bipolar needle electrode was repeatedly inserted through the perineal skin to detect the action potential of the external sphincter muscle. All insertions were within a depth of 5 mm. No anesthesia was used, to avoid muscle relaxation. The action potential of each external sphincter muscle was amplifired and displayed on the oscilloscope. Where required, the electromyograph was recorded on a film or a recording paper.

The degree of external sphincter muscle development was estimated by two methods. One was the so-called "external sphincter score." This name refers to the total number of examined points where the action potential of the external sphincter muscle could be picked up. In this method, a full mark would be 25 points, meaning that action potential could be picked up in all 25 points examined. The other method was by making a "distribution map of the external sphincter muscle." This is done by connecting the point at which the action potential could be picked up, as shown in Fig. 4.

In ten patients (seven with low- and three with high-type anomalies), an electromyographic examination was carried out repeatedly at an average interval of 5.3 months to check the development of the external sphincter muscle against body growth.

Results

External Sphincter Muscle Score. In patients with low-, intermediate-, and high-type anomalies, the scores were 18.3 ± 5.2, 12.7 ± 6, and 13.4 ± 6.6, respectively. These results indicate that the development of the external sphincter muscle of patients with intermediate- and high-type anomalies were more impaired than those of patients with low-type anomalies. But a wide standard deviation in each group indicated that the degree of development of this muscle varied in each case. Thus, the score in the case of a high-type anomaly was not necessarily poorer than that of a low-type anomaly. Excellent scores of over 20 points were demonstrated in four out of 23 patients with a high-type anomaly examined. Two out of those four patients were classified as having rectovesical fistulae (Fig. 2).

Distribution Map. Figure 3 shows the percentage of a detectable action potential of the external sphincter muscle at each point examined. The percentage was calculated by the formula, $P = (Cap/Ce) \times 100$; that is, the percentage *(P)* equals 100 times the number of cases in which action potential was detected *(Cap)*, divided by the number of cases examined *(Ce)*.

In over half of the low-type anomalies, the external sphincter muscle was distributed in an area 10 mm in width and 10 mm in ventodorsal length. However, in half of the intermediate- and high-type anomalies, the muscle was distributed in a limited area with a width of no more than 5 mm.

The skin mark on the perineum did not always indicate the center of distribution of the external sphincter muscle. A discrepancy between the skin mark and muscle distribution appeared in 21 out of 82 cases (25.9%) examined. An asymmetrical distribution of this muscle along the midline (Fig. 4c) was observed in 11

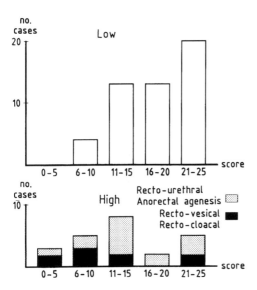

Fig. 2. Distribution of the external sphincter score in low- and high-type anomalies

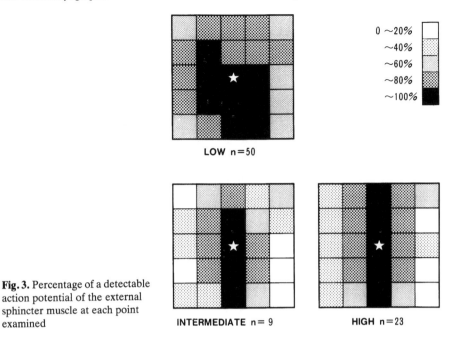

Fig. 3. Percentage of a detectable action potential of the external sphincter muscle at each point examined

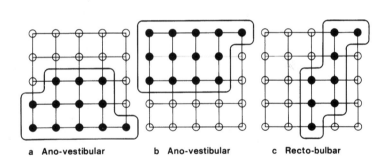

Fig. 4a–c. Discrepancy between skin marks and muscle distribution. **a** Dorsal deviation; **b** ventral deviation; **c** asymmetrical along the midline

cases (13.6%), and a difference in ventodorsal direction appeared in 10 cases (12.3%). Ventral deviation (when the muscle is located anteriorly to the skin mark, as shown in Fig. 4b) was observed in three cases, and dorsal deviation (Fig. 4a) was seen in seven cases.

Development of External Sphincter Muscle. An increase of the external sphincter score was documented in every case examined, thereby confirming that the development of the external sphincter muscle accompanied bodily growth. The score increase for low- and high-type anomalies at an average interval of 5.3

months was +1.9/25 and +3.7/25, respectively. One patient with a high-type anomaly showed a 5-point increase at an interval of 5 months.

Discussion

There have been many conflicting reports about the degree of development of the external sphincter muscle in anorectal malformations. Bryndorf and Madsen (1959/1960) observed that though the external sphincter muscle was present, it was deformed in a U shape. Stephens and Smith (1971c) stated that because the muscle fibers present at the perineum were quite thin and superficial, they could not be expected to function as sphincter muscles. However, Bill (1958) and Kiesewetter and Nixon (1967) reported that the external sphincter muscle was apparently present even in patients with anorectal malformations. Yokoyama et al. (1985) did serial sections on some examples of autopsied specimens and demonstrated that striated muscles were present in the locality of external sphincter muscle. They stated that those muscles not fragmentary were to be disregarded. Pena (1982) also reported that there was a lump of muscle complex even in the patients with high-type anorectal malformations.

The electromyographic examinations performed prior to the anorectoplasty showed the relatively abundant distribution of the external sphincter muscle at perineum around the dimple. Even in about half of the intermediate- and high-type anomalies, action potential of the external sphincter was able to be picked up in an area 5 mm in width and 10 mm in ventodorsal length. These muscles should not be disregarded in an anorectoplasty operation.

Furthermore, the increase in amplitude of the action potential of external sphincters was observed to synchronize with the increase in intra-abdominal pressure accompanying the young patients' crying. This means that where there was no agenesis of the sacrum, the reflex tract between the pelvic floor and the external sphincter muscle through the sacral spine (Porter 1962; Molander and Frenckner 1983) was completely normal. These findings could be interpreted as suggesting that the external sphincter muscles can provide postoperative fecal continence if they are preserved around the newly constructed anus.

Stephens and Smith (1971a) maintained that the muscle component capable of providing fecal continence was the puborectal muscle. The present research does not provide grounds for contesting the puborectal muscle's place as the most important factor in rectal control. However, as with the development of the external sphincter, the development of the puborectal muscle is also impaired to some degree in anorectal malformation. The electromyographic examination of the external sphincter muscle revealed that its development was good enough to provide fecal continence in half of even high-type anorectal malformations. It is therefore reasonable in operative repair to try to preserve both of these muscles as completely as possible and obtain the best fecal continence that the preserved integrity of these muscles can provide.

Two additional findings important for preserving the external sphincter in anorectal repair were obtained by electromyographic examinations. First, perineal appearance alone (the dimple or pigmentation, for instance) should not dictate the exact place where a new anus is constructed because there was found to be some discrepancy between skin marks and actual distribution of the sphincter muscle. Preoperative detection by electromyography and electric stimulation performed during anorectoplasty are strongly recommended for the purpose of preserving the external sphincter muscles. And, secondly, sequential electromyographic examinations demonstrated that the development of external sphincter muscles accompany normal bodily growth. In cases in which external sphincters distribute in a limited area at the perineum, repeated electromyographic examinations might provide useful information for deciding on an adequate chance for an anorectoplasty in which these muscles could be preserved.

Conclusions

Preoperative electromyographic examination was extremely useful in determining the exact location and degree of development of the external sphincter muscles. The electromyographic examinations showed the relatively abundant distribution of the external sphincter muscle at the perineum even in high-type anomalies. All the results, obtained by electromyographic examinations, lead to the conclusion that preserving both of the puborectal muscle and external sphincter muscles should be the chief consideration in the operation of the patients with an anorectal malformation.

References

Bill AH Jr (1958) Pathology and surgical treatment of "imperforated anus". JAMA 166:1429–1432
Bryndorf J, Madsen CM (1959/1960) Ectopic anus in the female. Acta Chir Scand 118:466–478
Kiesewetter WB, Nixon HH (1967) Imperforate anus I. Its surgical anatomy. J Pediatr Surg 2:60–68
Molander M-L, Frenckner B (1983) Electrical activity of the external anal sphincter at different ages in childhood. Gut 24:218–221
Pena A (1982) Posterior sagittal anorectoplasty: important technical considerations and new applications. J Pediatr Surg 17:796–811
Porter NH (1962) A physiological study of the pelvic floor in rectal prolapse. Ann Coll Surg Engl 31:379–404
Santulli TV, Kiesewetter WB, Bill AH (1970) Anorectal anomalies; a suspected international classification. J Pediatr Surg 5:281–287
Stephens FD, Smith ED (1971a) Ano-rectal malformations in children. Year Book Medical, Chicago, p 239
Stephens FD, Smith ED (1971b) Ano-rectal malformations in children. Year Book Medical, Chicago, pp 133–159
Stephens FD, Smith ED (1971c) Ano-rectal malformations in children. Year Book Medical, Chicago, pp 42–43, 68
Yokoyama J, Hayashi A, Ikawa H, Hagane K, Sanbonmatsu T, Endo M, Katsumata K (1985) Abdomino-extended sacroperineal approach in high-type anorectal malformation and a new operative method. Z Kinderchir 40:141–157

Diagnosis of Hirschsprung's Disease by Anorectal Manometry

A. Nagasaki[1], K. Sumitomo[1], T. Shono[2], and K. Ikeda[2]

Summary

Anorectal manometry was performed in 48 Japanese children with Hirschsprung's disease and 61 normal children. The resting pressure of the rectum and anal canal was not significantly different between these groups of subjects. The frequency of rhythmical contractions of the anal canal of patients was significantly lower than for the normal subjects, but the frequencies overlapped considerably. Therefore, the frequency is an inadequate indicator for identifying these patients.

Conventional manometry elicited a distinct rectoanal relaxation reflex from 90% of the normal children, and the rate increased to 98% when indistinct reflexes were regarded as positive. Indistinct reflexes often occur in neonates, possibly because the constriction of the anal canal is weak. However, when prostaglandin $F_{2\alpha}$ was intravenously administered during the examination, all ambiguous reflexes became distinct.

Of patients with Hirschsprung's disease, 4% had a distinct reflex and 19% an atypical one. Most of the atypical reflexes were regarded as being artifacts and were mostly attributed to distension by a balloon. In these patients, the reflex was abolished in case of examination with electric stimulation or stimulation with cold water, procedures which do not dilate the rectum. Moreover these atypical reflexes did not fit the criteria for the normal rectoanal relaxation reflex prepared by the Japan Study Group of Pediatric Intestinal Manometry. The use of electric stimulation, cold water, or intravenously administered prostaglandin $F_{2\alpha}$ improves reliability of the conventional anorectal manometry. A clear and accurate definition of the normal reflex should aid in excluding the atypical reflex.

Zusammenfassung

Bei 48 Kindern mit Hirschsprung-Krankheit und 61 gesunden Kindern in Japan wurden anorektale Manometrien durchgeführt. Der Ruhedruck im Rektum und Analkanal war nicht signifikant verschieden in beiden Gruppen. Die Häufigkeit der rhythmischen Kontraktionen des Analkanals war signifikant niedriger bei Kindern mit M. Hirschsprung als bei gesunden Kindern, jedoch zeigten beide Gruppen beträchtliche Überlappungen. Daher ist die Häufigkeit der rhythmischen Kontraktionen kein geeigneter Parameter zur Identifizierung der Kinder mit M. Hirschsprung.

Die konventionelle Manometrie ergab einen spezifischen rektoanalen Erschlaffungsreflex bei 90% der gesunden Kinder und diese Zahl wuchs auf 98% an, wenn unspezifische Reflexe mit einbezogen wurden. Unspezifische Reflexe werden häufig bei Neugeborenen beobachtet, möglicherweise weil die Konstriktion des Analkanals noch schwach ausgeprägt ist. Wenn jedoch während der Untersuchung Prostaglandin $F_{2\alpha}$ intravenös verabreicht wurde, wurden aus den unspezifischen Reflexen spezifische.

---

[1] Department of Surgery, Fukuoka Municipal Children's Hospital, 2-5-1 Tojin-machi, Chuo-ku, Fukuoka 810, Japan
[2] Department of Pediatric Surgery, Faculty of Medicine, Kyushu University, 3-1-1 Maidashi, Higashi-ku, Fukuoka 812, Japan

4% der Kinder mit M. Hirschsprung wiesen einen spezifischen, 19% einen atypischen Reflex auf. Die meisten atypischen Reflexe wurden als Artefakte durch die Balloninflation angesehen. Bei diesen Patienten wurde der Reflex aufgehoben, wenn die Untersuchung mittels Elektrostimulation oder Stimulation mit kaltem Wasser erfolgte, Verfahren, bei denen es zu keiner Dilatation des Rektums kommt. Außerdem stimmten diese atypischen Reflexe nicht mit den Kriterien des normalen rektoanalen Erschlaffungs-Reflexes der Japan Study Group of Pediatric Intestinal Manometry überein. Die Verwendung von Elektrostimulation, kaltem Wasser oder von i.v. verabreichtem Prostaglandin $F_{2\alpha}$ erhöht die Zuverlässigkeit der konventionellen anorektalen Manometrie. Eine klare und exakte Definition des normalen Reflexes muß den atypischen Reflex ausschließen.

Résumé

48 enfants atteints de maladie de Hirschsprung et 61 enfants sains ont été soumis à une manométrie anorectale. La pression de repos dans le rectum et le canal anal ne présentait pas de différence significative dans les deux groupes. La fréquence des contractions rythmiques du canal anal était significativement moins grande chez les enfants atteints de la maladie de Hirschsprung que chez les autres mais les deux groupes présentaient malgré tout des recoupements importants. C'est pourquoi la fréquence des contractions ne saurait constituer un paramètre fiable pour identifier les patients atteints de la maladie de Hirschsprung.

La manométrie conventionnelle montra un réflexe de relâchement recto-anal spécifique chez 90% des enfants sains, ce pourcentage atteignant même 98%, compte tenu des réflexes non spécifiques. On note souvent des réflexes non spécifiques chez les nouveaux-nés, du fait peut-être d'une constriction du canal anal encore peu prononcée. Si, pendant l'examen, il est procédé à une injection intraveineuse de prostaglandine F2 alpha, les réflexes non spécifiques se transforment en réflexes spécifiques.

Dans 4% des cas d'enfants atteints de la maladie de Hirschsprung on observa un réflexe spécifique et dans 19% des cas un réflexe atypique. La plupart des réflexes atypiques furent considérés comme étant des artéfacts dus au gonflement du ballon. Dans ces derniers cas, il y a eu disparition totale du réflexe lors de l'examen avec électrostimulation ou stimulation à l'eau froide, ces deux procédures n'entraînant pas de dilatation du rectum. D'autre part, ces réflexes atypiques ne correspondaient pas aux critères du réflexe de relâchement recto-anal normal établis par le Japan Study Group of Pediatric Intestinal Manometry.

L'électrostimulation, l'eau froide ou l'injection intraveineuse de prostaglandine F2 alpha augmentent la fiabilité de la manométrie anorectale conventionnelle. La définition précise du réflexe normal exige l'exclusion du réflexe atypique.

Introduction

When the rectum of a normal subject is distended by means of a balloon, the anal canal dilates, leading to a drop in intraluminal pressure (Gowers 1887). This is known as the "rectoanal relaxation reflex". In patients with Hirschsprung's disease, distension of the rectum fails to relax the anal canal, and there is no fall in the pressure (Schnaufer et al. 1967; Lawson and Nixon 1967). The anorectal manometry used to diagnose Hirschsprung's disease is based on this difference in the rectoanal relaxation reflex.

Anorectal manometry is not always diagnostic, as the reflex is not consistently present in neonates or even in normal infants (Holschneider et al. 1976; Ito et al. 1977) and is not absent in all patients affected with the disease (Meunier et al.

1978; Davis et al. 1981). On the other hand, some researchers (Bowes and Kling 1978; Tamate et al. 1984) have considered this method to be completely diagnostic.

The present study was an attempt to clarify causes which abolish the reflex in normal children or produce the reflex in patients and thereby to improve the manometric diagnosis of Hirschsprung's disease. Supplemental measures which aid in the diagnosis are presented.

Materials and Methods

The series comprised 48 Japanese children with Hirschsprung's disease. The ages ranged from 1 day to 7 years. All these patients were admitted to the Department of Pediatric Surgery of Kyushu University Hospital during the period from 1975 to 1986. Of these 48, 13 had undergone colostomy, and 7 were of the long-segment type in which aganglionosis extended to the small intestine. The control group comprised 61 subjects admitted to our department during the same period but without abnormal defecation. Here, the ages ranged from 2 days to 5 years.

Before the examination, a glycerin enema was given, and 100 mg/kg chloral hydrate was used for sedation when infants were not cooperative. The pressure was measured by the water-filled open-tip method with an LPU-0.1 transducer (Toyo Baldwin) coupled with a polygraph 360 system (NEC San-Ei). First, the resting pressure in the anorectum and the frequency of rhythmical contractions of the anal canal were recorded by the pull-through method using an 8-F polyvinyl tube with a side hole 1 mm in diameter. The rectoanal relaxation reflex was examined by the balloon distension method. When the reflex was atypical, the reflex was reexamined by administering electric stimulation under direct current of 1 ms and 20–30 V with 30 Hz (Nagasaki et al. 1984a) or 2–3 ml cold water at 4°C (Nagasaki et al. 1989) in place of distension with a balloon. Prostaglandin $F_{2\alpha}$ (Sumitomo et al. 1986b) was also given intravenously in a dose of 0.08 µg/kg per minute during the examination of some of the children.

Data here are expressed as means ± SD; statistical analysis was in terms of Student's t test. Levels lower than $P = 0.05$ were considered to be significant.

Results

Normal Children

In normal children, the mean resting pressure was 7.0 ± 2.9 cm H_2O in the rectum and 28.8 ± 14.8 cm H_2O in the anal canal. The mean frequency of contractions of the anal canal was 11.4 ± 1.9 per minute. When the normal subjects were divided into three groups according to age – neonate group (< 28 days), infant group (< 1 year), and young children group (> 1 year) – there was no significant age-related difference found in these parameters (Table 1). The rectoanal relaxation reflex

Table 1. Anorectal manometry of normal children and children with Hirschsprung's disease

	Number of patients	Rectal pressure (cm H$_2$O)	Anal-canal pressure (cm H$_2$O)	Frequency of rhythmic wave (contractions/min)	Appearance of reflex (%)[a]
Normal children	61	7.0 ± 2.9	28.8 ± 14.8	11.4 ± 1.9 ⎤[d]	90 (98)
Neonates	19	6.7 ± 1.5	29.7 ± 15.0	11.0 ± 1.4	73 (94)
Infants	29	8.1 ± 2.6	27.9 ± 16.4	12.0 ± 2.1	96 (100)
Young children	13	5.0 ± 2.8	29.6 ± 11.0	12.0 ± 2.0 ⎦	100
Hirschsprung's disease	48	9.8 ± 4.3	31.7 ± 14.6	8.6 ± 1.5 ⎦	4 (23)
Neonates	18	10.0 ± 3.6	27.4 ± 14.3	8.3 ± 1.8	0 (17)
Infants	21	9.1 ± 4.1	30.3 ± 10.3 ⎤[c]	8.5 ± 1.2	5 (21)
Young children	9	13.1 ± 6.0	56.0 ± 16.8 ⎦	9.7 ± 1.7	11 (44)
Without colostomy	35	9.6 ± 3.7	28.9 ± 11.2 ⎤[b]	8.6 ± 1.7	3 (17)
With colostomy	13	9.2 ± 4.3	38.5 ± 15.1 ⎦	8.4 ± 1.2	8 (38)
Long segment	7	11.2 ± 4.3	30.0 ± 21.2	8.9 ± 0.9	0 (29)

[a] Figures in parentheses represent appearance rate including atypical reflexes
[b] $P < 0.05$
[c] $P < 0.02$
[d] $P < 0.001$

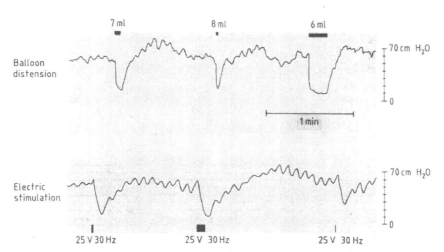

Fig. 1. Rectoanal relaxation reflex in a normal infant produced by balloon distension (atypical reflex) and by electric stimulation (typical reflex)

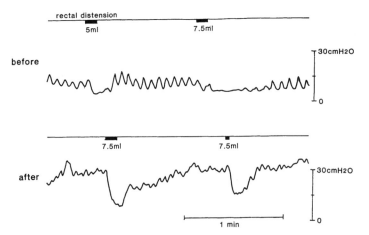

Fig. 2. Rectoanal relaxation reflex before and after administration of prostaglandin $F_{2\alpha}$ in a normal infant

was demonstrated in all subjects of the young children group and infant group, except for a suckling infant whose reflex was irregular. Of five neonates, one was unresponsive, and the reflex was obscure in the remaining four. Reexamination with electric stimulation could induce a typical reflex in the infant whose reflex was irregular (Fig. 1). In the neonate who failed to respond to the balloon test, a small reflex was induced in case of a reexamination with a combination of intravenous prostaglandin $F_{2\alpha}$. Prostaglandin $F_{2\alpha}$ also aided in eliciting evident reflexes from the four neonates (Fig. 2). A typical reflex was seen when these neonates were reexamined by the balloon method after several days. The first examination induced a distinct normal reflex in 59 of 61 normal subjects with the aid of electric stimulation or prostaglandin $F_{2\alpha}$. Reexamination improved the ratio to 100%.

Patients with Hirschsprung's Disease

In children with Hirschsprung's disease, the resting pressure was 9.8 ± 4.3 cm H_2O in the rectum and 31.7 ± 14.6 cm H_2O in the anal canal. These values were not significantly different from findings in the normal children (Table 1). Anal canal pressure in the young children group was significantly higher than that for either of the other two groups ($P < 0.02$). The anal-canal pressure for children undergoing colostomy was significantly higher than that for the other children ($P < 0.05$). In cases of the long-segment type, the resting pressure did not differ from that for the entire group of patients.

The frequency of contractions of the anal canal was 8.6 ± 1.5 per minute, a finding significantly lower than that for normal children ($P < 0.001$). There was no significant difference among the groups or in terms of the absence or presence of a colostomy.

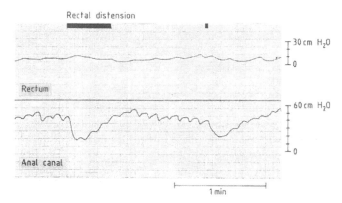

Fig. 3. Typical rectoanal relaxation reflex in a child with Hirschsprung's disease

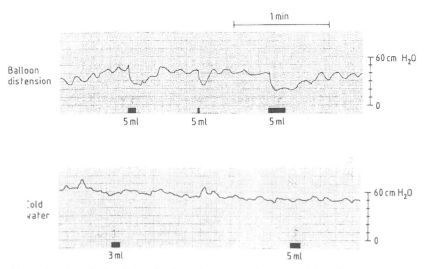

Fig. 4. Atypical rectoanal relaxation reflex by balloon test and absence of the reflex by cold water in a child with Hirschsprung's disease

The balloon distension elicited a typical rectoanal relaxation reflex in two subjects (Fig. 3) and an atypical reflex in nine. The reflex, although atypical, was induced more frequently in the young children group than in the other two age groups and in patients with a colostomy more frequently than in those without it. However, there was no evidence suggesting that the test elicited the reflex from patients with the long-segment type. Electric stimulation and cold water were used to examine two each of the nine children who responded to the examination with an atypical reflex, but no reflex could be induced (Fig. 4). Eventually, the reflex was positive in two and pseudopositive in five children, although in these patients neither electric stimulation nor cold water was applied.

Discussion

To improve the manometric diagnosis of Hirschsprung's disease a number of points must be noted. First, other factors, such as the resting pressure of the rectum and the anal canal and the frequency of rhythmical contractions of the anal canal, should be used for reference. Secondly, diagnostic criteria for the positive response of the reflex should be clearly defined. And, thirdly, the technique to record the reflex should be improved.

We consider the rectoanal relaxation reflex to be the best indicator for the diagnosis of Hirschsprung's disease because there is no significant difference in the resting pressure between normal children and patients, and although the anus contracts more frequently in normal children than in patients, the frequencies overlapped over a wide range.

The normal reflex, as defined by the Japan Study Group of Pediatric Intestinal Manometry (Nagasaki et al. 1978), is as follows:

1. The anal-canal pressure begins to drop 1–3 s after distension of the rectum and is gradually restored to the resting level.
2. The duration of fall in the anal-canal pressure is essentially invariable, independent of the duration of rectal distension.
3. The pressure drops at least three times in a single examination.
4. The anal-canal rhythmical waves should be observable.

These criteria aid in distinguishing an atypical reflex from the normal reflex. However, the test may elicit a reflex to meet the criteria from patients with Hirschsprung's disease, but most such reflexes are artifacts, likely due to distention of the balloon. The situations under which such artifacts are produced are illustrated in Fig. 5. To avoid such artifacts, we used electric stimulation or stimulation with cold water. As described elsewhere (Nagasaki et al. 1984a), in normal children, either electric stimulation or administration of cold water can induce a clear rectoanal relaxation reflex similar to one induced by the balloon method. In the present study, the electric stimulation induced a typical reflex in one in which the the balloon method induced an irregular reflex. The electric stimulation and cold water failed to elicit any reflex in four of nine patients (two by each method) in whom the conventional balloon method induced an atypical reflex. In these four, the inflated balloon might have dilated not only the lumen of the rectum but also the anal canal, thereby lowering the pressure. When there is no concomitant dilation of the anal canal, only relevant changes in the anal-canal pressure are obtained. Frenchner (1983) estimated the same mechanism using electric stimulation.

Some neonates may not respond to the test, even if they are apparently normal. Of the normal neonates examined in the present study, one had no reflex at all and four only a small fall in anal-canal pressure. In most of these five, the pres-

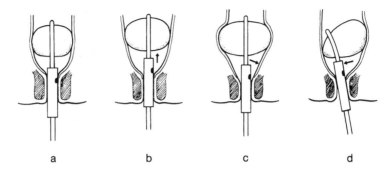

Fig. 5a–d. The causes of false-positive reflex. **a** Normal study. **b** Withdrawing of the probe into the rectum. **c** Overdistension of the rectum. **d** Distorted dilatation of the balloon

sure of the anal canal was low. In patients subjected to radical surgery for an imperforate anus, the higher the resting pressure of the anal canal was, the more frequent was the reflex (Nagasaki et al. 1984b). Prostaglandin $F_{2\alpha}$ exerts action directly on the smooth muscle of the intestine, increases the contraction force (Bennet 1970) and facilitates the rectoanal relaxation reflex (Sumitomo et al. 1986a). In subjects who responded to the conventional manometric examination with an ambiguous reflex, the reflex became evident when the examination was carried out in combination with an intravenous administration of prostaglandin $F_{2\alpha}$. On the other hand, Sumitomo et al. (1986b) reported that in patients with Hirschsprung's disease and an ambiguous reflex, administration of prostaglandin $F_{2\alpha}$ either failed to enhance the reflex or abolished it. Therefore, the use of drugs to increase contraction of the smooth muscles, for example prostaglandin $F_{2\alpha}$, can make distinct the presence or absence of the reflex, leading to improvement of the manometric diagnosis of Hirschsprung's disease.

The immaturity of ganglion cells in the intestine may possibly be responsible for the absence of the reflex seen in neonates (Ito et al. 1977). In addition, the present study suggested that the weak contraction of the anal canal may also be responsible.

References

Bennett A (1970) Control of gastrointestinal motility by substances occurring in the gut wall. Rend R Gastroenterol 2:133–142
Bowes KL, Kling S (1979) Anorectal manometry in premature infants. J Pediatr Surg 14:533–535
Davis MRQ, Cywes S, Rode H (1981) The manometric evaluation of the rectosphincteric reflex in total colonic aganglionosis. J Pediatr Surg 16:660–663
Frenchner G (1983) Rectal myenteric nerve plexus stimulation in Hirschsprung's disease and in healthy children. Z Kinderchir 38:396–399
Gowers WR (1987) The automatic action of the sphincter ani. Proc R Soc Lond 26:77–84

Holschneider AM, Kellner E, Streibl P, Sippell G (1976) The developement of anorectal continence and its significance in the diagnosis of Hirschsprung's disease. J Pediatr Surg 11:151–156

Ito Y, Donahoe PK, Hendren WH (1977) Maturation of the rectoanal response in premature and perinatal infants. J Pediatr Surg 12:477–482

Lawson JON, Nixon HH (1967) Anal canal pressure in the diagnosis of Hirschsprung's disease. J Pediatr Surg 2:544–552

Meunier P, Marechar JM, Mollare P (1978) Accuracy of the manometric diagnosis of Hirschsprung's disease. J Pediatr Surg 13:411–415

Nagasaki A, Ikeda K, Suzuki H, Katsumata K (1978) Criteria for judgement of positive rectoanal reflex. Rinsho To Kenkyu 55:3545–3550 (in Japanese)

Nagasaki A, Ikeda K, Suita S, Sumitomo K (1984a) Induction of the rectoanal reflex by electric stimulation. A diagnostic aid for Hirschsprung's disease. Dis Colon Rectum 27:598–601

Nagasaki A, Ikeda K, Hayashida Y, Sumitomo K, Sameshima S (1984b) Assessment of bowel control with anorectal manometry after surgery for anorectal malformation. Jpn J Surg 14:229–234

Nagasaki A, Ikeda K, Sumitomo K (1989) Recto-anal reflex induced by H_2O thermal stimulation. Dis Colon Rectum (in press)

Schnaufer L, Talbert JL, Reid NCRW, Tobon F, Schuster MM (1967) Differential sphincteric studies in the diagnosis of ano-rectal diagnosis of childhood. J Pediatr Surg 2:538–543

Sumitomo K, Ikeda K, Nagasaki A (1986a) The effect of autonomic drugs and prostaglandin $F_{2\alpha}$ on the rectoanal inhibitory reflex. Z Kinderchir 41:35–38

Sumitomo K, Ikeda K, Nagasaki A (1986b) The use of prostaglandin $F_{2\alpha}$ and scopolamine-N-butylbromide in anorectal manometric diagnosis. Z Kinderchir 41:435–438

Tamate S, Shiokawa C, Yamada C, Takeuchi S, Nakahira M, Kadowaki H (1984) Manometric diagnosis of Hirschsprung's disease in the neonatal period. J Pediatr Surg 19:285–288

Problems in Diagnosis of Hirschsprung's Disease by Anorectal Manometry

J. Yokoyama, T. Kuroda, H. Matsufugi, S. Hirobe, S. Hara, and K. Katsumata

Summary

The purpose of this study is to analyze the results of anorectal manometry and to evaluate the merits and disadvantages of this technique for the diagnosis of Hirschsprung's disease. Studies were performed in 268 patients with constipation, including 95 cases of Hirschsprung's disease. It is concluded from the results that Hirschsprung's disease can be confidently diagnosed by manometric studies. If the studies are performed carefully with a suitable probe, reliability is over 95%. Manometry is the most useful method to differentiate Hirschsprung's disease from other conditions, such as extremely short segment aganglionosis, colonic stenosis, and idiopathic megacolon.

Zusammenfassung

In dieser Arbeit sollen die Ergebnisse der anorektalen Manometrie und deren Vor- und Nachteile bei der Diagnose des M. Hirschsprung analysiert werden. Elektromanometrische Untersuchungen wurden bei 268 Kindern mit Obstipation durchgeführt, unter denen sich 95 mit Hirschsprung-Krankheit fanden. Aus den Ergebnissen wird der Schluß gezogen, daß der M. Hirschsprung durch die manometrischen Untersuchungen zuverlässig diagnostiert werden konnte. Wenn die Untersuchungen sorgfältig und mit einer geeigneten Sonde durchgeführt werden, liegt die Zuverlässigkeit dieser Methode bei über 95%. Die Manometrie ist die am besten geeignete Methode, den M. Hirschsprung von anderen pathologischen Veränderungen wie ein extrem kurzes aganglionäres Segment, eine Kolonstenose oder ein idiopathisches Megakolon abzugrenzen.

Résumé

Cette étude a pour but d'analyse l'évaluation de la manométrie anorectale et la comparaison de ses avantages et ses inconvénients dans le diagnostic de la maladie de Hirschsprung. Nous avons pratiqué des examens électro-manométriques sur 268 enfants atteints de constipation et avons décelé 95 cas de maladie de Hirschsprung. Les résultats indiquent que ces examens ont permis de diagnostiquer cette affection de façon fiable. A la condition d'une pratique très minutieuse de ces examens et de l'utilisation d'une sonde adéquate, la fiabilité de cette méthode est de plus de 95%. La manométrie est la méthode de choix à la frontière entre la maladie de Hirschsprung et les autres pathologies voisines telles qu'un segment aganglionnaire très court, une sténose du côlon ou encore un mégacôlon idiopathique.

Department of Pediatric Surgery, School of Medicine, Keio University, 35 Shinanomachi, Shinjuku-ku, Tokyo 160, Japan

Introduction

Lawson and Nixon (1967) demonstrated for the first time that the rectoanal reflex which is observed in normal infants was not recognized in Hirschsprung's disease. Since 1971 we have experienced 268 cases of infants and children with constipation and have performed measurement of the rectoanal reflex a total of 368 times. Rectoanal manometric measurement has become a useful technique to confirm organic disorders in constipated children and is widely used at present. The purpose of this report is to analyze the results of our manometric study and to evaluate the merits and disadvantages of this technique for the diagnosis of Hirschsprung's disease.

Materials and Methods

Studies were performed on 268 cases with constipation at Keio University Hospital between 1973 and 1986. The subjects ranged in age from newborn infants to children of 14 years. Six cases of premature babies and ten cases which needed to be differentiated from Hirschsprung's disease at their bedside were included in this series (Table 1). Also, we experienced 29 cases of Hirschsprung's disease with

Table 1. Results of rectoanal reflex analysis of cases with abnormal bowel function

Results	Number of cases in final diagnosis	Number of cases showing negative rectoanal reflex at initial examination	Number of cases in which examination was repeated
Constipation	157	3[a]	3
Hirschsprung's disease	95	95	18
Premature babies	6	6[a]	6
Septic cases	3	3	
Suspected NID	2	2	
Severe colonic stenosis after necrotizing enterocolitis	1	1	
Rectal stenosis after perforation	1 } 10	1 } 10[a]	10
Meningocele	1	1	
Unknown enterocolitis	1	1	
Aplasia of thyroid	1	1	
Total	268	114	37

[a] Cases showing atypical response at the initial examination of the rectoanal reflex

colostomy in whom the rectoanal reflex was also measured. However, 2–3 weeks after initial examination their rectoanal reflex was normal. Manometry was performed to confirm the diagnosis in one patient with colostomy whose diagnosis of Hirschsprung's disease had been made in another hospital. Surprisingly, this patient showed the presence of rectoanal reflex.

We devised our original instrument for manometry in 1971; this consists of a stainless-steel tube with a double lumen. The advantage of this probe is the sensitive sensor, a 50-micron polyurethane membrane, near the tip of the probe on the wall of the outer lumen. Our preliminary basic experimental studies demonstrated that a polyurethane membrane with a width of 50 microns has a particular elasticity to detect tiny pressure changes in the anal canal. Details of this probe and the method of measurement are presented by Yokoyama et al. (this volume).

For measurement of the rectoanal reflex, rectal stimulation with a balloon is done four times. For the initial three times, the rectum is stimulated for 2–3 s; for the last one, the stimulus is prolonged. Following each stimulus, a 2- to 3-s delay in response is recorded before the pressure starts to fall. The pressure then returns to baseline after 10–13 s in normal cases. Even if the stimulus is prolonged with the distended balloon, this pressure pattern is not altered. When a typical pressure response after stimulation is recorded four times in succession, the patient is diagnosed as having a normal rectoanal reflex, in other words, a positive rectoanal reflex.

Results

Rectoanal Reflex in Constipated Children

Hirschsprung's disease was ruled out in 154 of 268 cases with functional constipation by the first manometry. However, three cases did not show a typical rectoanal reflex as defined above at the initial examination, but repeated examination did demonstrate a normal reflex. All 157 cases showing the presence of the rectoanal reflex showed no clinical problem after the examination (Table 1). In 18 out of the 95 cases of Hirschsprung's disease, the rectoanal reflex was equivocal at the initial examination. We repeated the test two or three times and finally concluded that there was no reflex in these cases. In all cases without the rectoanal reflex, aganglionosis was confirmed by histochemical examination or histological studies.

There were six premature babies in whom the rectoanal reflex at the initial examination was absent. However, they showed a normal reflex 2–3 weeks after the initial examination (Fig. 1).

Demonstration of a narrow segment by barium enema is an available method to diagnose Hirschsprung's disease. However, a narrow segment is not always seen in every case of Hirschsprung's disease, especially in the case of short-segment aganglionosis. We experienced a case of short-segment aganglionosis in which the rectoanal reflex was not demonstrable, and no narrow segment was visible by barium enema (Fig. 2).

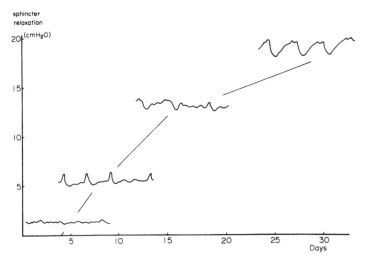

Fig. 1. Sphincter relaxation in a premature infant. At the initial examination, the normal response for rectal stimulation by balloon was absent, however the normal response was seen 3 weeks after the initial study

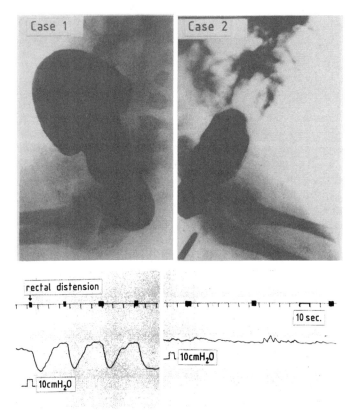

Fig. 2. The narrow segment was not demonstrated by barium enema in either case 1 or 2, however the normal response to the distended rectal balloon was not recognized in case 2

Table 2. Results of rectoanal reflex analysis of cases with bowel obstruction

Results	Number of cases	Rectoanal reflex	Number of cases in which examination was repeated
Colon atresia	1	Positive	
Volvulus of small intestine	1	Positive	
Rectal atresia	1	Positive	5
Meconium ileus	1	Positive	
Segmental dilatation of sigmoid	1	Positive	
Total	5		5

Table 3. Aplasia of thyroid (hypothyroidism)

Clinical signs and parameters	1 Jan	28 Mar	22 Apr	1 May	27 May	Aug.	Oct.
		Colostomy →		Administration of thyroid drugs →			
Convulsions	++	++		+++	(−)	(−)	(−)
Abdominal distension	++	++		+	(−)	(−)	(−)
^{131}I-labeled T_3 (25%–37%)			23	19.2	21.2	31.7	34
^{125}I-labeled T_4 (5–13 dl)			1.1	1.9	6.7	7.9	8.9
Thyroid-stimulating hormone ($<10\,\gamma$/ml)				330			
T (90–220 µg/dl)				15			
Rectoanal reflex			(−)				++

There were ten cases which needed to be differentiated from Hirschsprung's disease at their bedside (Table 1). These ten cases showed unexpected results; they demonstrated the absence of a rectoanal reflex even though the bowels were nonaganglionic. Three of these were septic, and two cases were suggestive of disease similar to neuronal intestinal dysplasia (NID; Puri and Nixon 1977; Schärli and Meier-Ruge 1981) from the pathological findings. Other cases included diseases such as aplasia of the thyroid, sigmoidal stenosis after necrotizing enterocolitis, lower rectal stenosis after perforation of rectum, sacral meningocele, and severe chronic enterocolitis.

In cases with sepsis, the resting anal-canal pressure was extremely low, which may account for the absence of a rectoanal reflex. On the other hand, five cases which had bowel obstruction, such as colon atresia, volvulus of the small intestine, rectal atresia, meconium ileus, and segmental dilatation of the sigmoid showed the typical reflex (Table 2).

Table 4. Final results of rectoanal reflex analysis and final diagnosis of the patients

			Final diagnosis
Presence of rectoanal reflex	163		
	157		Constipation
	6		Premature babies
Absence of rectoanal reflex	105		
	95		Hirschsprung's disease
		3	Septic cases
		2	Suspected NID
		1	Severe colonic stenosis after necrotizing enterocolitis
	10	1	Rectal stenosis after perforation
		1	Meningocele
		1	Unknown enterocolitis
		1	Aplasia of thyroid

The case of thyroid aplasia involved marked abdominal distension and constipation after birth. Because of suspicion of Hirschsprung's disease colostomy was done at a local hospital and without pathological examination. The patient showed no rectoanal reflex before the colostomy. The constipation and abdominal distension did not improve after the construction of colostomy. From the results of endocrine examination, aplasia of the thyroid was diagnosed. After the administration of a thyroid drug, the abdominal distension improved, and the rectoanal reflex appeared (Table 3).

Table 4 demonstrates the overall results of rectoanal reflex analysis and final diagnosis of the constipated patients. In 100% of the patients who showed a rectoanal reflex, Hirschsprung's disease could be excluded clinically. Of the 105 patients who showed absence of the reflex, 95 were diagnosed as having Hirschsprung's disease. The ten other cases were originally misdiagnosed. This misdiagnosis in the three septic cases was caused by hypotonicity of resting pressure in the anal canal. Severe scaring in the colon and rectum after the infection may be another cause of misdiagnosis. As for the case with meningocele, sacral denervation is suspected. The other cases included aplasia of the thyroid, two cases of suspected NID, and severe chronic enterocolitis of unknown cause. Therefore, the diagnostic rate of certain Hirschsprung's disease was 85% of those cases showing a negative reflex. However, the overall reliability of 94% compares very favorably with that of other reports (Table 4).

Rectoanal Reflex in Hirschsprung's Disease with Colostomy

Eight cases of Hirschsprung's disease with colostomy demonstrated the rectoanal reflex. The first case with colostomy showing rectoanal reflex was transferred to

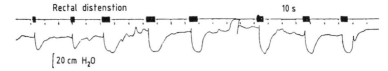

Fig. 3. A case of Hirschsprung's disease with colostomy and a typical rectoanal reflex in spite of pathological demonstration of aganglionic bowel

us from another hospital for evaluation. The case showed a typical rectoanal reflex in spite of pathological demonstration of aganglionic bowel (Fig. 3). From this experience, we examined the rectoanal reflex in cases of Hirschsprung's disease after construction of colostomy. Reflex patterns were normal in most cases. Some cases, however, showed a prompt fall in pressure after rectal stimulation, without any time delay.

Discussion

Rectoanal manometry is a physiological examination. If the patients are not physiologically normal, as in sepsis or hypothyroidism, the results of the examination in these patients might be affected. Therefore, it is very important to evaluate the condition of the patient before the examination, and the manometric study should be performed only on those displaying normal physiological conditions. In this condition, even a tiny pressure change in the anal canal may be detected.

Our original probe (Fig. 4) has a membrane sensor made of 50-micron-thick polyurethane with particular elasticity to detect anal-canal pressure changes. We think it not possible to detect pressures of internal sphincter and external sphincter separately because the anal-canal pressure is dependent primarily on sustained activity of the internal sphincter, not on voluntary tonus of the external one.

From our experimental studies (Yokoyama et al., this volume), electrical activity of the internal sphincter was seen to correlate well with changes in anal-canal pressure. Our probe with a single-membrane sensor can accurately detect the tiny pressure changes of the anal canal surrounded by the internal sphincter.

In our manometric study, the overall reliability in constipated patients was 94%. Aaronson and Nixon (1972) found it easier to exclude Hirschsprung's disease (90.8%) than to confirm its presence (74.3%) in their manometric study, and their overall diagnostic reliability was 85%. Meunier and Mollard (1976) also performed a manometric study on 140 cases of constipated patients using the open-tip method, and their rate of misdiagnosis was only 4%.

In the following, we will discuss those cases which showed unexpected responses. There were 19 cases which showed unexpected responses at the initial examination of rectoanal reflex (Table 1). These cases included three cases of constipation, six of premature babies, three of sepsis, two of suspected NID, and one

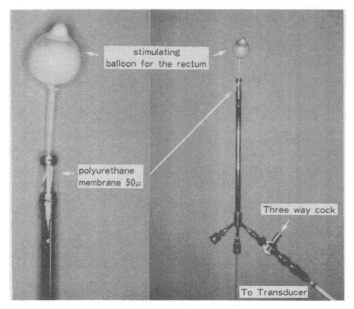

Fig. 4. Our original probe used to measure the rectoanal reflex

each of severe colonic and rectal stenosis, meningocele, severe unknown enterocolitis, and thyroid aplasia.

Premature babies in whom we could not initially record a rectoanal reflex ranged from 1.3 to 1.8 kg in weight and from 35 to 38 weeks in gestation. These premature babies showed the rectoanal reflex when they reached 39 weeks of gestation. However, low weight and early gestation does not always cause the absence of a rectoanal reflex. We experienced two other cases of premature babies of 31 and 33 weeks of gestation, respectively, who showed a rectoanal reflex. All three babies with sepsis died without showing a rectoanal reflex. Their resting anal-canal pressure was distinctly lower than the normal range in the control group. The low anal-canal pressure may have been responsible for the absence of the reflex.

The case of congenital aplasia of the thyroid had convulsion and vomitings with abdominal distension after birth. Colostomy was done in another hospital following a suspicion of Hirschsprung's disease. After transference to our hospital and examination of his thyroid function, the patient was diagnosed as having congenital agenesis of the thyroid. Manometric study performed before treatment did not show rectoanal reflex. After he was treated with thyroid hormone for 5 months, however, the reflex appeard.

We can not clearly explain the reason why these 19 cases did not demonstrate the rectoanal reflex at the initial examination in spite of the fact that they had ganglionic bowels. However, we may safely say that in premature babies, imma-

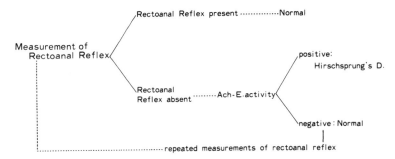

Fig. 5. New diagnostic method for constipated patients

turity of ganglion cells may be responsible. While, in spetic cases and in the case of thyroid agenesis, functional disorders in the neurotransmission system due to original diseases may be responsible for the absence of the rectoanal reflex. In the cases of severe colonic and rectal stenosis, the anal canal was deformed with scaring after infection. There have been several discussions of the pathophysiology of NID. Further evaluation of the pathology and physiology of NID is needed, as they are not yet clear.

We had eight cases with colostomy which showed rectoanal reflex in spite of the operative diagnosis of Hirschsprung's disease. Several factors may elicit the rectoanal reflex. One is an artifact due to dilation by the balloon of the narrowing of the anal canal caused by colostomy. Another factor is a change in hormonal circumstances or metabolism of neurotransmitters in the rectal wall after the construction of colostomy, because no further stool passes through the distal colon and rectum. In any event, we still do not clearly understand this unexpected phenomena. However, we should be cautious in deciding whether the rectoanal reflex is pesent in cases with colostomy.

At our institution, the diagnosis of Hirschsprung's disease is done first by manometric study with reference to the findings of barium enema. Cases which show a typical rectoanal reflex at initial examination are followed clinically as functional constipation. Concerning the cases that show no rectoanal reflex, repetitive study is performed in 1–2 weeks (Fig. 5). Meanwhile, suction biopsy of the rectal mucosa is conducted for histochemical staining (Meier-Ruge 1974). As stated earlier, we do not record a rectoanal reflex as being positive unless the typical fall of pressure can be demonstrated four times successively in a recording.

We conclude that Hirschsprung's disease can be excluded confidently by manometric study. If the study is performed carefully with a suitable probe, the reliability of this method is over 95%. We would like to conclude by emphasizing, finally, that manometry is the most useful method to differentiate Hirschsprung's disease from other conditions, such as extremely short segment aganglionosis, congenital ilial atresia, colonic stenosis, and idiopathic megacolon.

References

Aaronson I, Nixon HH (1972) A clinical evaluation of anorectal pressure studies in the diagnosis of Hirschsprung's disease. Gut 13:138–146

Lawson JON, Nixon HH (1967) Anal canal pressures in the diagnosis of Hirschsprung's disease. J Pediatr Surg 2:544–552

Meier-Ruge W (1974) Hirschsprung's disease: its etiology, pathogenesis and differential diagnosis. Curr Top Pathol 59:131–179

Meunier P, Mollard P (1976) Manometric studies of anorectal disorders in infancy and childhood: an investigation of the physiopathology of continence and defecation. Br J Surg 63:402–407

Puri P, Nixon HH (1977) Neuronal colonic dysplasia: an unusual association of Hirschsprung's disease. J Pediatr Surg 12:681–685

Schärli AF, Meier-Ruge W (1981) Localized and disseminated forms of neuronal intestinal dysplasia mimicking Hirschsprung's disease. J Pediatr Surg 16:164–170

Anorectal Manometry After Ikeda's Z-Shaped Anastomosis in Hirschsprung's Disease

A. Nagasaki[1], K. Sumitomo[1], T. Shono[2], and K. Ikeda[2]

Summary

The intraluminal pressure of the rectum and anal canal were measured in patients with Hirschsprung's disease before and after Ikeda's Z-shaped anastomosis, and the association of the pressure with postoperative capability of fecal continence was assessed.

Radical operation did not alter rectal pressure but did decrease anal-canal pressure. Rhythmical anal contractions increased in frequency until a normal level was attained. The rectoanal relaxation reflex became distinct with time, and 45% of patients eventually attained the reflex after operation.

In patients who postoperatively attained satisfactory fecal continence or, at least, only soiling, resting pressure in the anorectum and the frequency of rhythmical anal-canal contractions were similar to those for normal children. The rectoanal relaxation reflex was induced in 58% of the former and 27% of the latter. In patients with postoperative constipation, the intraluminal resting pressure of the anorectum was elevated without the relaxation reflex response. In patients with incontinence, the pressure of the anal canal was low, without a reflex response. These findings indicate that the high and low values of the resting pressure of the anal canal are responsible for constipation and incontinence, respectively, and that the presence of rectoanal relaxation reflex may represent one aspect of a normal defecation function.

Zusammenfassung

Der intraluminale Druck in Rektum und Analkanal wurde bei Patienten mit M. Hirschsprung vor und nach Z-Anastomose nach Ikeda gemessen und der Zusammenhang zwischen Druck und postoperativer Kontinenz bestimmt.

Eine radikale Operation veränderte den Druck im Rektum nicht, führte aber zu einer Drucksenkung im Analkanal. Die Häufigkeit der rhythmischen Kontraktionen des Analkanals nahm zu, bis normale Werte erreicht waren. Mit der Zeit bildete sich ein ausgeprägter rektoanaler Erschlaffungsreflex aus, der bei 45% der Patienten endgültig nach der Operation erreicht wurde. Bei Kindern, die postoperativ ausreichende Kontinenz oder zumindest nur Stuhlschmieren erreichten, waren der Ruhedruck im Anorektum und die Frequenz der rhythmischen Kontraktionen des Analkanals denen normaler Kinder ähnlich. Bei 58% der Kinder wurde ein rektoanaler Erschlaffungsreflex und bei 27% wurden rhythmische Kontraktionen des Analkanals herbeigeführt. Bei Kindern mit postoperativer Obstipation war der intraluminale Ruhedruck erhöht, und es fehlte der Erschlaffungsreflex. Bei Kindern mit postoperativer Inkontinenz fand sich ein niedriger Ruhedruck im Analkanal, und es fehlte ebenfalls der Erschlaffungsreflex. Die Ergebnisse sprechen dafür, daß ein hoher oder ein niedriger Ruhedruck verantwortlich für Ob-

---

[1] Department of Surgery, Fukuoka Municipal Children's Hospital, 2-5-1 Tojin-machi, Chuo-ku, Fukuoka 810, Japan
[2] Department of Pediatric Surgery, Faculty of Medicine, Kyushu University, 3-1-1 Maidashi, Higashi-ku, Fukuoka 812, Japan

stipation bzw. Inkontinenz sind und daß das Vorliegen eines rektoanalen Erschlaffungsreflexes nur ein Aspekt der normalen Defäkationsfunktion ist.

Résumé

La pression intraluminale dans le rectum et le canal anal a été mesurée chez des patients atteints de maladie de Hirschsprung avant et après une anastomose en Z d'après Ikeda et on a ainsi déterminé le degré de relation entre pression et continence post-opératoire.

Une opération radicale ne modifie pas la pression dans le rectum mais la fait baisser dans le canal anal. La fréquence des contractions rhythmiques dans le canal anal augmente jusqu'a l'obtention de données normales. A la longue, un net réflexe de relâchement recto-anal a pu être être obtenu définitivement dans le cas de 45% des patients opérés. Pour les enfants ayant retrouvé une continence post-opératoire suffisante ou du moins ne présentant plus qu'un spotting, on note une pression de repos anorectale et une fréquence des contractions rythmiques du canal anal comparables à celles des enfants sains. Pour 58% des enfants on a obtenu un réflexe de relâchement recto-anal et pour 27% des contractions rythmiques du canal anal. Chez les enfants atteints de constipation post opératoire, la pression intraluminale au repos avait augmenté et il n'y avait pas de réflexe de relâchement. Dans le cas des enfants présentant une incontinence post-opératoire, la pression au repos dans le canal anal était basse et il n'y avait pas non plus de réflexe de relâchement. Les résultats indiquent nettement qu'une pression trop élevée ou trop basse provoque la constipation ou l'incontinence et que la présence d'un réflexe de relâchement recto-anal n'est qu'un aspect de la fonction normale de défécation.

Introduction

It is of interest to know whether the rectoanal relaxation reflex appears after radical operation in patients with Hirschsprung's disease, and whether its appearance is associated with postoperative fecal continence. Only a few reports have dealt with this subject (Frenckner and Lindstrom 1983; Iwai et al. 1983; Kasai et al. 1977; Nagasaki et al. 1980; Schuster et al. 1963; Suzuki et al. 1970).

We performed anorectal manometry in infants with Hirschsprung's disease, before and after Ikeda's Z-shaped anastomosis (Ikeda 1967) − a modified Duhamel's procedure − and investigated the relationship between postoperative fecal continence and the findings of anorectal manometry.

Materials and Methods

Clinical assessment of fecal continence and anorectal manometry were performed in 46 patients who had undergone Ikeda's Z-shaped anastomosis. In 27 patients who were operated upon during the period from 1975 to 1986 at the Department of Pediatric Surgery, Kyushu University, the examination was carried out before surgery and 1−2, 6, 12, and 24−36 months after the operation. In 19 patients who had undergone the Z-shaped anastomosis before 1975, only postoperative assessment of fecal continence and anorectal manometry could be done. All the patients were over 3 years of age at the time of assessment of fecal continence.

The water-filled open-tip method, as described elsewhere (Nagasaki et al. 1984, 1987), was used for the manometry. The control group consisted of 61 normal children (Nagasaki et al. 1987).

The results are given in terms of means ± SD. Student's t test was used for statistical analysis. Levels lower than $P = 0.05$ were considered statistically significant.

Results

Anorectal Manometry Before and After Surgery

The mean preoperative resting pressure of the rectum was 9.5 ± 3.9 cm H$_2$O. The operative treatment did not essentially alter the pressure (Table 1). Anal-canal pressure was 31.6 ± 13.2 cm H$_2$O preoperatively but dropped to 22.1 ± 10.8 cm H$_2$O ($P < 0.02$) 2–3 months after operation, and this level was maintained for 2–3 years. The mean frequency of rhythmical contractions of the anal canal was 8.1 ± 1.6 per minute preoperatively, and there was an increase to 10.1 ± 1.9 per minute 1–2 months after surgery ($P < 0.01$). No change occurred thereafter.

Before operation, the rectoanal relaxation reflex was clear in two of the 39 cases and atypical (irregular or small) in seven. The remaining 30 patients did not respond to the stimulation. When examined 1–2 months after operation, the clear reflex was not demonstrable in any patient, but five patients did have an atypical reflex. Subsequently, the reflex became distinct with time. A marked reflex was obtained in 45% of patients 2–3 years after the surgery. The rate increased to 80% when those with an atypical reflex response were included (Fig. 1).

Table 1. Anorectal manometry of children with Hirschsprung's disease before and after Ikeda's Z-shaped anastomosis

	Number of patients	Rectal pressure (cm H$_2$O)	Anal-canal pressure (cm H$_2$O)	Frequency of rhythmic wave (contractions/min)	Appearance of reflex (%)[a]
Control	61	7.0 ± 2.9	28.8 ± 14.8	11.4 ± 1.9	90 (98)
Preoperative	39	9.5 ± 3.9	31.6 ± 13.2 [b]	8.6 ± 1.6 [c]	8 (23)
Postoperative					
1–2 months	36	10.3 ± 5.6	22.1 ± 10.8	10.1 ± 1.9	0 (13)
6 months	26	9.1 ± 3.5	21.1 ± 6.4	10.3 ± 1.4	15 (53)
1 year	25	9.2 ± 3.2	25.8 ± 13.3	10.6 ± 1.9	24 (64)
2–3 years	20	8.5 ± 3.5	21.0 ± 8.0	10.9 ± 1.4	45 (80)

[a] Figures in parentheses represent appearance rate including atypical reflexes
[b] $P < 0.02$
[c] $P < 0.01$

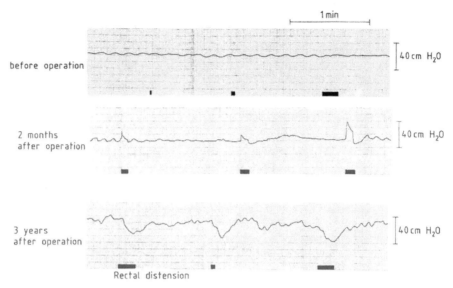

Fig. 1. Rectoanal relaxation reflex before, 2 months after, and 3 years after operation in a boy with Hirschsprung's disease

Correlation with Fecal Continence

In patients with normal continence after surgery, the resting pressure of the anorectum and the frequency of rhythmical contractions of the anal canal were not significantly different from those for normal children (Table 2). The rectoanal relaxation reflex was induced in 58% of the patients (Fig. 2).

In constipated patients, the mean resting pressures in the rectum and anal canal were 12.6 ± 4.1 cm H_2O and 47.5 ± 19.6 cm H_2O, respectively, and were sig-

Table 2. Postoperative continence and anorectal manometry after Z-shaped anastomosis for Hirschsprung's disease

	Number of patients	Rectal pressure (cm H_2O)	Anal-canal pressure (cm H_2O)	Frequency of rhythmic wave (contractions/min)	Appearance of reflex (%)[a]
Control	61	7.0 ± 2.9[b]	28.8 ± 14.8[b]	11.4 ± 1.9	90 (98)
Good continence	24	6.6 ± 5.6	31.6 ± 13.5	12.2 ± 1.7	58 (79)
Constipation	6	12.6 ± 4.1	47.5 ± 19.6	12.7 ± 1.6	0 (50)
Soiling	11	4.4 ± 5.2	25.3 ± 13.4	11.7 ± 2.2	27 (63)
Incontinence	5	6.0 ± 2.1	17.0 ± 5.6	12.0 ± 0.9	0 (40)

[a] Figures in parentheses represent appearance rate including atypical reflexes
[b] $P < 0.05$

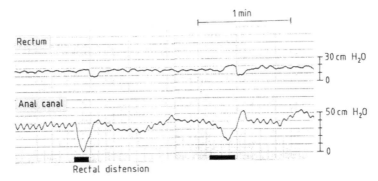

Fig. 2. Rectoanal relaxation reflex in a 3-year-old girl with normal continence 2 years after surgery for Hirschsprung's disease

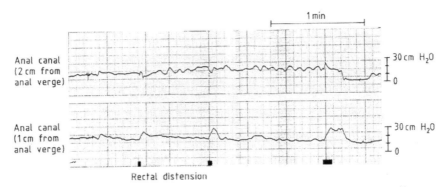

Fig. 3. Absent rectoanal relaxation reflex in a 7-year-old boy with fecal incontinence 7 years after surgery for Hirschsprung's disease

nificantly higher than those determined in normal children ($P < 0.05$). No distinct rectoanal relaxation reflex was elicited from any patient, and an atypical reflex was observed only in three (50%).

In patients with problems of fecal soiling, the resting pressure at the anorectum and the frequency of anal contractions were identical with those for normal children. The reflex was elicited from three (27%).

In the cases of incontinence, the resting pressure of the anal canal was 17.0 ± 5.6 cm H_2O, lower than that for normal children ($P < 0.05$). No clear reflex was induced in any of these patients, but an atypical reflex was induced in two (40%) (Fig. 3).

Discussion

The rectoanal relaxation reflex is absent in Hirschsprung's disease (Schnaufer et al. 1967; Lawson and Nixon 1967). This absence has been regarded as one of factors causing constipation in patients with this disease (Schnaufer et al. 1967). The constipation can be overcome after appropriate radical operation. Whether the rectoanal relaxation reflex can be acquired after the operation, and whether the postoperative capability of fecal continence varies depending on the presence or absence of the reflex, have been discussed (Kasai et al. 1977; Nagasaki et al. 1980; Frenckner and Lindstrom 1983).

After Z-shaped anastomosis, the rectal pressure was not reduced, yet the anal-canal pressure decreased. The operation that we used removed two-thirds of the posterior half of the internal anal sphincter muscle, thereby reducing anal-canal strain. The reduction may have led to a postoperative decrease in anal-canal pressure. Postoperatively, frequency of the rhythmical anal contractions increased to levels similar to levels in normal children, but the reasons for this are not well understood. The rectoanal relaxation reflex became distinct with time. Eventually the test elicited the reflex from 45% of patients 2–3 years after the operation. In the literature, this rate varies with the researcher (Frenckner and Lindstrom 1983; Iwai et al. 1983; Kasai et al. 1977; Nagasaki et al. 1980; Schuster et al. 1963; Suzuki et al. 1970). Here, differences in surgical mode and in criteria for positive response may play some role. The postoperative rectoanal reflex is usually atypical even if it is attained; therefore, it is difficult to determine the extent of positive reflex. We used the criteria prepared by the Japan Study Group of Pediatric Intestinal Manometry (Nagasaki et al. 1989) as a reference. According to Holschneider (1982), based on manometric observation, about 30% of patients surgically treated by the method of Swenson, Duhamel, Soave, or Rehbein attained the reflex.

The postoperative appearance of the reflex, as described above, may be the result of the capability of transmission of stimuli from the colon to the sphincter muscles. The radical operation to remove the aganglionic portion leads to a connection of the anal canal with the colon, containing normal intramural neural innervation. However, even if the muscles of the colon are linked to those of the anus, nerve fibers arising in the colon may not necessarily enter the sphincter muscle and achieve control of the muscle. The reflex has been attained in many subjected to Lynn's rectal myectomy (Suzuki et al. 1970; Nagasaki et al. 1980), thereby suggesting that the elimination of the anal spasm is essential for appearance of the reflex.

In patients who attained a normal fecal continence, the resting pressure in the anorectum and the frequency of the anal-canal contractions were similar to those in normal children. The rectoanal relaxation reflex was elicited from 58% of the patients.

In patients with constipation, both rectal and anal-canal pressures were higher than those for normal children, without a distinct rectoanal relaxation reflex. It is not certain whether the increased anal-canal pressure caused the constipation. According to Hung (1975), however, partial sphincterotomy may alleviate constipation because the excessive strain of the internal anal sphincter is partly involved in the etiology.

In patients with incontinence after operation, the anal-canal resting pressure was lower than that for normal children, perhaps became of a weak constriction strength of the anal canal. Postoperative incontinence in patients with an imperforate anus (Nagasaki et al. 1984; Iwai et al. 1979) and other disease (Arhan et al. 1984; Hiltunen 1985) is also associated with low anal-canal pressure. The rectoanal relaxation reflex could not be elicited from patients with postoperative incontinence. It has been reported that the rectoanal relaxation reflex alone is insufficient for evaluating functions related to defecation, and that contraction of the external anal sphincter is essential for the prevention of incontinence (White et al. 1973). The sensation of fecal evacuation and rectal compliance are also involved in fecal continence. However the presence of the rectoanal relaxation reflex invariably represents a normal defecating function. In cases of an imperforate anus, the reflex has frequently been attained when the patients attained normal defecation function after operation (Nagasaki et al. 1984; Iwai et al. 1979; Taylor et al. 1973). While the meaning of rhythmical contractions of the anal canal remains to be clarified, these contractions were frequently absent in patients with a severe incontinence.

References

Arhan P, Faverdin C, Devroed G, Pierre-Kahn A, Scott H, Pellerin D (1984) Anorectal motility after surgery for spina bifida. Dis Colon Rectum 27:159–163
Frenckner B, Lindstrom O (1983) Ano-rectal function assessed by manometric and electromyography after endorectal pull-through for Hirschsprung's disease. Z Kinderchir 38:101–104
Hiltunen KM (1985) Anal manometric findings in patients with anal incontinence. Dis Colon Rectum 28:925–928
Holschneider AM (1982) Hirschsprung's disease. Hippokrates, Stuttgart, p 240
Ilung WT (1975) Experience with a modification of Duhamel-Grob-Martin operation for the treatment of Hirschsprung's disease. Surgery 77:680–686
Ikeda K (1967) New technique in the surgical treatment of Hirschsprung's disease. Surgery 61:503–508
Iwai N, Ogita S, Kida M, Fujita Y, Majima S (1979) A clinical and manometric correlation for assessment of postoperative continence in imperforate anus. J Pediatr Surg 14:538–543
Iwai N, Hashimoto K, Kaneda H, Tsuto T, Yanagihara J, Majima S (1983) Manometric assessment of anorectal pressure in Hirschsprung's disease after Rehbein's operation with and without anorectal myectomy. Z Kinderchir 38:316–319
Kasai M, Suzuki H, O'hi R, O'htomo S (1977) Rectoplasty with posterior triangular colonic flap – a radical new operation for Hirschsprung's disease. J Pediatr Surg 12:207–211
Lawson JON, Nixon HH (1967) Anal canal pressure in the diagnosis of Hirschsprung's disease. J Pediatr Surg 2:544–552
Nagasaki A, Ikeda K, Suita S (1980) Postoperative sequential anorectal manometric study of children with Hirschsprung's disease. J Pediatr Surg 15:615–619
Nagasaki A, Ikeda K, Hayashida Y, Sumitomo K, Sameshima S (1984) Assessment of bowel control with anorectal manometry after surgery for anorectal malformation. Jpn J Surg 14:229–234
Nagasaki A, Sumitomo K, Shono T, Ikeda K (1989) Diagnosis of Hirschsprung's disease by anorectal manometry. Prog Pediatr Surg 24:40–48
Schnaufer L, Talbert JL, Reid NCRW, Tobon F, Schuster MM (1967) Differential sphincteric studies in the diagnosis of ano-rectal diagnosis of childhood. J Pediatr Surg 2:538–543
Schuster MM, Hendrix TR, Mendeloff AI (1963) The internal anal sphincter response: Manometric studies on its normal physiology, neural pathways and alteration in bowel disorders. J Clin Invest 42:196–207

Suzuki H, Watanabe K, Kasai M (1970) Manometric and cineradiologic studies on anorectal motility in Hirschsprung's disease before and after surgery operation. Tohoku J Exp Med 102:69–80

Taylor I, Duthie HL, Zachary RB (1973) Anal continence following surgery for imperforate anus. J Pediatr Surg 8:497–503

White JJ, Suzuki H, El Shafie M, Kumar APM, Haller JA, Schnaufer L (1973) Physiologic responses of the ano-rectal sphincters in children with incontinence and constipation problems. Am Surg 39:95–100

Motility of the Anorectum After the Soave-Denda Operation

Y. Morikawa[1], H. Matsufugi[2], S. Hirobe[2], J. Yokoyama[2], and K. Katsumata[2]

Summary

A total of 82 patients were assessed by rectal manometry after operation for Hirschsprung's disease according to the Soave-Denda technique. A positive rectoanal reflex was obtained in 32 cases (39%), whereas the remaining 50 cases (61%) did not exhibit a rectoanal reflex. Among the children examined, 72% showed normal rhythmic activity of the anorectum. Anorectal function tended to increase over the years, 90% having good continence 10 years or more after operation. Patients who encountered postoperative complications had poor continence since such complications may have damaged the levator and sphincter muscles.

Zusammenfassung

82 Kinder mit M. Hirschsprung wurden mittels rektaler Manometrie nach Soave-Denda-Operation nachuntersucht. Bei 32 Fällen (39%) fand sich ein positiver rektoanaler Reflex, während ein solcher bei den restlichen 50 Kindern (61%) nicht nachweisbar war. 72% der Kinder wiesen normale rhythmische Aktivität des Anorektums auf. Die anorektale Funktion zeigte eine Tendenz, sich über die Jahre zu verbessern, wobei 90% der Kinder eine gute Kontinenzleistung nach 10 Jahren und später hatten. Patienten mit postoperativen Komplikationen zeigten schlechte Kontinenz, da diese Komplikationen die Levator- und Sphinktermuskulatur beschädigt hatten.

Résumé

82 enfants atteints de la maladie de Hirschsprung ont été examinés par manométrie rectale après une opération selon Soave-Denda. Dans 32 cas, soit 39%, on a trouvé un réflexe recto-anal positif alors que chez les 50 autres enfants, soit 61%, on n'a pas pu prouver la présence d'un réflexe recto-anal. L'activité rythmique de l'anorectum était normale chez 72% des enfants. La fonction anorectale tendait nettement à s'améliorer à la longue et 90% des enfants avaient retrouvé une bonne continence 10 ans et plus après l'intervention. Les patients chez lesquels des complications post-opératoires étaient survenues présentaient aussi une mauvaise continence, ces complications ayant atteint le releveur et la musculature du sphincter.

---

[1] Department of Pediatric Surgery, Urawa City Hospital, 2460 Mimuro, Urawa, Saitama 336, Japan
[2] Department of Pediatric Surgery, School of Medicine, Keio University, 35 Shinanomachi, Shinjuku-ku, Tokyo 160, Japan

Introduction

The postoperative function of the anorectum has been well documented, mainly by qualitative assessment (Kelly 1969), and operative results in Hirschsprung's disease have been reported for years. Although most patients acquire a satisfactory anorectal function after radical treatment, data indicate that some patients have a poor anorectal function. Moreover, there is the possibility that differences in surgical procedure may yield different results on the postoperative anorectal function. Since the Soave-Denda endorectal pull-through operation can be considered noninvasive to the pelvic plexus, with a complete excision of the aganglionic segment, one should expect superior results using this technique.

Making an objective evaluation of the anorectal function in growing children can be difficult, especially in younger infants. Therefore, it seems important that the assessment be programmed in terms of the subject's development. To make these evaluations quantitative, a manometric technique has been adopted for years. In this chapter, we describe our technique and the results of analysis in relation to the clinical assessment over our 15 years of experience.

Materials and Methods

A total of 82 cases of Hirschsprung's disease were assessed after various periods following radical treatment using the KY rectal manometry probe. A water-filled double-lumen catheter with a membrane sensor of polyurethane was placed across the internal anal sphincter to detect changes in pressure. The inner lumen of the probe consists of a fine tube connected to the balloon for rectal stimulation. A detailed technique of manometry has been described elsewhere (Morikawa et al. 1979). The rectoanal reflex was registered as positive when a reproducible fall in pressure was obtained after at least three consecutive balloon stimulations with a certain latency. A pressure fall which did not meet this criterion but responded to rectal stimulation was considered an atypical reflex.

Rhythmic changes in the resting pressure of the anal canal were measured and counted as cycles per minute from the actual tracing. Some of the data were recorded in a data recorder (TEAC MR-10) and stored in an MT unit (TEAC MT-800) after analog to digital conversion for further evaluation. The power spectrum and the autocorrelation function of the wave form were obtained by fast Fourier transform (FFT) using a microcomputer (TEAC PS-85), with a sampling frequency of 5 Hz and 1024 data points.

Patients were also subjected to clinical assessment of the anorectal function in terms of rectal sensation, continence, and staining, using the modified Kelly code (Kelly 1969).

Patient Selection. Patients were operated on by the Soave-Denda endorectal pull-through method (Soave 1964; Denda 1966) upon diagnosis of Hirschsprung's disease, confirmed either by histology or manometry in combination with acetylcholinesterase histochemistry. They were divided into four groups according to the length of time since surgery. These were: group I, under 3 years (17 patients); group II, 3–7 years (34); group III, 7–10 years (20); and group IV, over 10 years (13). Most patients thus fell into groups of II or III (64%). Ages of patients for postoperative assessment ranged from 18 months to 19 years, with a median of 6 years and 7 months, and was generally associated with length of time since surgery.

Type of Treatment. Denda's technique was utilized with an endorectal pull-through approach, which is characterized by a primary anastomosis of colon pulled through to the anus and an excision of the muscle strip of the posterior wall of the rectal cuff down to the internal anal sphincter. The endorectal pull-through technique allows complete preservation of the pelvic plexus, and, in addition, Denda's technique can avoid possible stricture of the anus accompanying Soave's original nonsutured method. Most patients in the present series received a two-stage operation.

Statistics. A χ^2 test and Student's t test were used for statistical analysis in evaluating the rectoanal reflex and the rhythmic wave of the anorectal function after surgery.

Results

A positive rectoanal reflex was obtained in 32 cases (39%); a typical reflex was counted in 15 (18%) and an atypical reflex in 17 (21%) cases. In 50 cases (61%) a negative rectoanal reflex was revealed, in spite of careful manometric study (Table 1). Among the patients with over 7 years postoperative, 44% showed a positive reflex, and among those with under 7 years of postoperative course 37% did so. There was no significant difference between these two groups.

Rhythmic movement of the internal anal sphincter was measured in 71 cases, at various postoperative points. In 72% (51/71) of patients there was a normal pattern of rhythmic activity characterized by two major cycles. In 20 cases using the Soave-Denda technique, these rhythmic changes were not detected, although

Table 1. Rectoanal reflex: results

Rectoanal reflex	Number of patients (%)	
Positive	32	(39%)
Typical	15	(18%)
Atypical	17	(21%)
Negative	50	(61%)
Total	82	(100%)

some irregular pressure changes in lower frequencies were recorded. In 21 out of 22 cases (95.55%) with a positive rectoanal reflex, there was rhythmic activity of the anal canal, while 61% of cases with a negative reflex showed a rhythmic wave ($P<0.01$). The frequency of these rhythmic waves during the first 10 years after surgery was 10.19 ± 2.60 cpm, and this did not seem to fluctuate throughout the period. The frequency increased to 13.12 ± 1.97 cpm in the next 10 years ($P<0.01$; Fig. 1).

The power spectrum of pressure changes was computed by FFT in six patients. The analysis revealed two major peaks, which represent the maximal power of the basal slow wave and the rhythmic wave of the internal anal sphincter respectively (Fig. 2). The frequency of slow basal waves was about the same as in the nine nor-

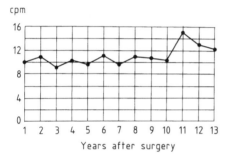

Fig. 1. Frequency of the rhythmic wave after the Soave-Denda procedure in the first 13 years following surgery

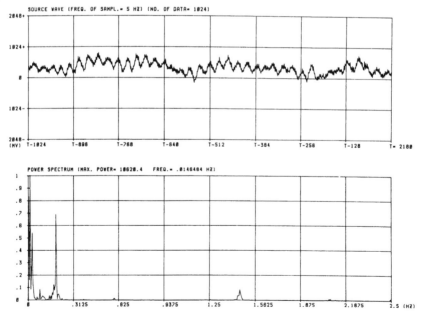

Fig. 2. Power spectrum of pressure changes of anal canal at resting state, obtained from a patient with positive rectoanal reflex

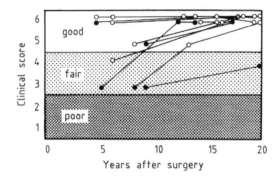

Fig. 3. Long-term follow-up study on postoperative anorectal function. *Open circles* indicate positive reflex; *closed circles*, negative reflex; a *dotted circle* equivocal reflex

Table 2. Constipation, rectal sensation, and the anorectal reflex

	Positive reflex	Negative reflex
Constipation		
None	86%	94%
Mild	7%	6%
Severe	7%	0%
Rectal sensation		
Always	79%	68%
Sometimes	21%	32%
None	0%	0%

mal controls, i.e., approximately 1.0 cpm. On the other hand, the mean frequency of maximal power of the rhythmic wave range was significantly lower than in controls (9.96 ± 2.96 cpm versus 14.55 ± 4.56 cpm; $P < 0.05$).

A long-term follow-up study was carried out on the rectoanal reflex, and the clinical score at various points from 5 to 20 years after surgery was determined. Figure 3 indicates the change in anorectal function, which tends to increase over time. In 40% (4/10) of cases the score was under 4 in the first 10 years; this is considered to be fair. All patients became socially functional and enjoyed their activities after the first 10-year period. In the following 10 years, 90% of cases were evaluated as good (score 5 or 6). The rectoanal reflex was positive in 44% of cases during postoperative years, including three cases with an atypical form of the reflex. The number of patients with a positive reflex increased with time, and 63% of them are positive 15 years after radical treatment.

There seemed to be no difference in constipation problems between reflex-positive and -negative patients (Table 2). A rectal sensation of oncoming stool was reported in 79% of the reflex-positive group and in 68% of the reflex-negative group.

Table 3. Postoperative anorectal function in patients with and without Hirschsprung's disease

	Hirschsprung's disease			Control[a]		
	3–7 years	7–10 years	Over 10 years	3–6 years	6–9 years	9–12 years
Defecation						
Over 3 per day	13.8%	19.0%	23.0%	0.4%	0.0%	0.0%
Over 2 per day	55.2%	23.8%	15.4%	5.5%	8.7%	15.2%
One in 2 days	27.6%	57.2%	54.3%	83.1%	73.3%	77.6%
One in 3 days	0.0%	0.0%	7.3%	10.6%	14.7%	6.2%
Less than 1 in 3 days	3.4%	0.0%	0.0%	0.4%	3.3%	1.0%
Rectal sensation						
None	6.0%	0.0%	0.0%	1.3%	1.3%	1.4%
Occasional	27.3%	15.0%	0.0%	7.6%	8.6%	4.6%
Always	66.7%	85.0%	100.0%	91.1%	90.1%	94.4%

[a] Data from Hayashi et al. (1985)

Defecation was frequent in the early postoperative period (Table 3). Bowel movements occurred more than twice a day (55.2%), and 13.8% of patients in group II had bowel movement more than three times a day. In group III, 57.2% were in the normal range, which seems to be that of a bowel movement once a day or once in 2 days, according to observation of normal controls. However, 23% of patients in group IV still passed stool more than three times a day.

A rectal sensation of oncoming stool was poor to some degree among those of the shortest postoperative course (see Table 2). Among group II patients, 6% had no rectal sensation, and 27.3% had occasional, and another 66.7% normal, rectal sensation. In group IV, no significant difference was observed in comparison to the normal controls.

Fecal incontinence of various degrees was seen in eight cases in group II, one in group III, and one in group IV. Their manometry revealed negative rectoanal reflex to any stimulation. Although patients classified in group I were incontinent in many cases, they were excluded from evaluation in the present study since normal bowel control is thought to be established after the age of 4 years. In grop II, 58% had normal continence, and the proportion of continent subjects increased with years after treatment. In group IV, 84.6% of patients were fully continent. Patients with a positive rectoanal reflex all had good fecal continence, however in spite of a negative reflex 63% had also good control.

Frequent staining (over one per week) occurred in group II (56%), and a marked improvement was seen in group IV (23%). Staining was more frequent (87%) among patients with a negative rectoanal reflex (Table 4).

Leakage and abscess formation have been documented as major postoperative complications of the Soave-Denda operation (Deodbar et al. 1973; Kleinhaus et al. 1979; Velcek et al. 1982). Small leakage and abscess were seen in 11 cases in

Table 4. Incontinence, staining, and the anorectal reflex

	Positive reflex	Negative reflex
Incontinence		
Over 2 per week	0	6 (19%)
Under 1 per week	0	4 (13%)
In case of diarrhea	3 (21%)	5 (16%)
None	11 (79%)	16 (52%)
Staining		
Over 2 per week	5 (36%)	16 (52%)
Under 1 per week	4 (28%)	11 (35%)
In case of diarrhea	0	1 (3%)
None	5 (36%)	3 (10%)

the present series (13%). A second operation was carried out in four cases. Among patients with fecal incontinence (excluding those with under 3 years after surgery), 63% had a history of leakage.

Discussion

Motility of the anorectum after colorectal surgery in children has been extensively investigated for years by many surgical institutions. Observations have been based upon clinical evaluations of anorectal function in terms of continence, rectal sensation, etc. (Soave 1977; Jordan et al. 1979; Kleinhaus et al. 1979). The manometric technique was first introduced into this field by Callaghan and Nixon (1964) for patients with constipation, and this tool was utilized for evaluating operative results of anorectal surgery in the field of pediatric surgery (Suzuki et al. 1970). Since those with Hirschsprung's disease are known to lack a rectoanal reflex, manometry has become a reliable diagnostic tool and has been utilized in many facilities. Moreover, the fact that patients who received the pull-through operation could have a rectoanal reflex, made the study of rectal pressure one of the modalities in evaluating the postoperative function of the anorectum in Hirschsprung's disease.

Appearance of the reflex after surgery was noted in 39% of cases in the present series, which is considerably high. Presence of the reflex did not seem to affect rectal sensation or constipation. On the other hand, incontinence and staining were significantly lower in patients with a positive reflex; this does not necessarily mean, however, that patients with a negative reflex always exhibit poor anorectal function.

The mechanism of the reflex after the pull-through operation is still obscure. The structures that give tone and motility to the anorectum are the complex of internal anal sphincter, external anal sphincter, pulled-through colon, and levator muscles. Most of these structures receive surgical manipulation to some degree, except the external anal sphincter. The upper two-thirds of the internal sphincter is excised with an aganglionic segment, and additional excision is made at its posterior part with a rectal cuff by the Soave-Denda technique. It is uncertain whether a rectoanal reflex after surgery is due directly to internal sphincter relaxation, however recent observations using the extradural electrode technique suggest that the rest of internal sphincter may not be responsible for the pressure fall in a patient who had a Soave-Denda operation (Morikawa and Sanbonmatsu 1986). A case in which a fall in pressure of the anal canal responded to rectal stimulation has been reported in a patient with Hirschsprung's disease who had had a colostomy (Morikawa et al. 1975). Similar change is known to occur after abdominoperineal correction of anorectal malformations even in the case of a patient with a high-type anomaly (Yokoyama et al. 1974). Yokoyama et al. 1974, 1985) speculated that a puborectal muscle and an inner circular muscle of the rectum play a significant role as a functional internal sphincter in the presence of the rectoanal reflex and continence after surgical treatment. Ihara and Takahira (1984) reported that an electrical stimulation to the sacral nerve could simulate a rectoanal reflex in the decerebrated dog. They observed that inhibition of electrical activity of the internal anal sphincter occurred, accompanied by a pressure fall after stimulation to the sacral nerve. It is conceivable that a muscular component of the anorectum other than the internal anal sphincter is responsible for the postoperative anorectal reflex in Hirschsprung's disease. The possibility of a newly pulled-through colon giving some nervous control to the internal anal sphincter seems very slim. However, these reflexes may be caused by relaxation of the pulled-through colon, according to the "intestinal law" (Bayliss and Starling 1899). This idea militates against the observation made by Ihara and Takahira (1984) who demonstrated a fall in tone of the anal canal when they divided the sacral nerve on both sides.

A rhythmic wave was observed in 72% of the cases. A relationship between these waves and anorectal function in each case is not clear, although their frequency tends to increase after the first 10 years of the postoperative period, which also sees an improvement of the clinical score.

FFT analysis revealed two major peaks of frequency in power-spectral density. A slow component of the peak is thought to be derived from a "minute rhythm" which may indicate a proper motility of the smooth muscle of pulled-through colon. The second peak, in a higher range of frequency, reflects rhythmic contraction of the internal anal sphincter which is significantly lower than that in controls. Morikawa et al. (1985, unpublished data) demonstrated that a rhythmic wave consists of different waves, and that the peak frequency in Hirschsprung's disease is low. Analysis of the autocorrelation function of these waves confirmed that there exists a certain dominant cycle.

Patients who experienced complications apparently had poor continence. Since these complications may have led to considerable damage to the levator and sphincter muscles, these structures seem to play an important role in producing a rectoanal reflex. Schuster et al. (1963) reported that a rectoanal reflex was not detected in any of their five cases after Swenson's procedure. A whole structure of rectum as a receptor is lost, and the continuity of the colon to the sphincter is broken by this operative method. In addition, a puborectal muscle and the pelvic plexus may be damaged to a certain extent, in contrast to the case with the Soave-Denda operation. Although there is a possibility that the mechanism of the postoperative rectoanal reflex may be different from that in the normal reflex, it seems reasonable that the appearance of a rectoanal reflex after surgery requires some continuity of the lower rectum to the internal sphincter by an intact puborectal muscle.

Further follow-up study needs to be done to determine whether there is a difference in the anorectal function among patients with differences in the unresected aganglionic segment.

Acknowledgement. The authors are grateful to Mrs. Kyoko Yasuda for her excellent assistance in preparing manuscript.

References

Bayliss WM, Starling EH (1899) The movement and innervation of the small intestine. J Physiol 24:99–143
Callaghan RP, Nixon HH (1964) Megarectum; physical observation. Arch Dis Child 39:153–157
Denda T (1966) Surgical treatment of Hirschsprung's disease: a modification of Soave procedure. Geka Shinryo 8:295–301
Deodbar M, Sieber WK, Kiesewetter WB (1973) A critical look at the Soave procedure for Hirschsprung's disease. J Pediatr Surg 8:249–254
Hayashi A, Ishida H, Kamagata S, Ueno S, Sugitani K, Murakoshi T, Katsumata K (1985) Late complications of Hirschsprung's disease and anorectal manometry. J Jpn Surg Soc 9:1290–1292
Ihara N, Takahira E (1984) Regulation of anal canal pressure as revealed by myoelectrical activity of internal anal sphincter. Jpn J Smooth Muscle Res 20:123–135
Jordan FT, Coran AG, Weintraub WH, Wesley JR (1979) An evaluation of the modified endorectal procedure for Hirschsprung's disease. J Pediatr Surg 14:681–685
Kelly JH (1969) Cineradiography in anorectal malformations. J Pediatr Surg 4:538–546
Kleinhaus S, Boley SJ, Sheran M, Sieber W (1979) Hirschsprung's disease: a survey of the members of the Surgical Section of the American Academy of Pediatrics. J Pediatr Surg 14:588–597
Morikawa Y, Sanbonmatsu T (1986) Change of anal canal pressure and electrical activity of the internal anal sphincter after electrical stimulation to the spinal cord. J Jpn Soc Pediatr Surg 22:351
Morikawa Y, Hayashi A, Ito Y, Namba S, Yokoyama J, Katsumata K (1975) Change in histochemistry and manometry following colostomy. Jpn J Smooth Muscle Res 11:204–205
Morikawa Y, Donahoe PK, Hendren WH (1979) Manometry and histochemistry in the diagnosis of Hirschsprung's disease. Pediatrics 63:865–871
Nagasaki A, Ikeda K, Suita S (1980) Postoperative sequential anorectal manometric study of children with Hirschsprung's disease. J Pediatr Surg 15:615–619
Schuster MM, Hendrix TR (1963) The internal anal sphincter response; manometric studies on its normal physiology, neural pathways, and alteration in bowel disorders. J Clin Invest 42:196–207
Soave F (1964) Hirschsprung's disease: a new surgical technique. Arch Dis Child 39:116–124
Soave F (1977) Long-term results of operative treatment in Hirschsprung's disease. Z Kinderchir 22:267–279

Suzuki H, Watanabe K, Kasai M (1970) Manometric and cineradiographic studies on anorectal motility in Hirschsprung's disease before and after surgical operation. Tohoku J Exp Med 102:69–80

Velcek FT, Klotz DH, Friedman A, Kottmeier PK (1982) Operative failure and secondary repair in Hirschsprung's disease. J Pediatr Surg 17:779–785

Yokoyama J, Ito Y, Namba S, Morikawa Y, Takuhashi M, Ogata T, Yokoyama S, Katsumata K (1974) Postoperative manometric assessment of high type anomaly of the anorectal malformations. J Jpn Soc Pediatr Surg 10:192

Yokoyama J, Hayashi A, Ikawa H, Hagane K, Sanbonmatsu T, Endo M, Katsumata K (1985) Abdomino-extended sacroperineal approach in high-type anorectal malformation − and a new operative method. Z Kinderchir 40:151–157

Anorectal Motility After Rectal Myectomy in Patients with Hirschsprung's Disease

R. Ohi[1] and K. Komatsu[2]

Summary

Anorectal manometric studies were performed 42 times in 13 patients with rectal myectomy and 137 times in 49 cases treated by the PTCF method. The resting pressure of the anal canal was found to be lowered just after the operation and remained at levels lower than those in normal controls and in patients with rectal myectomy. This fact was attributed to the resection of the muscle layer in the anal canal. On the other hand, the resting pressure of the anal canal in patients undergoing the PTCF method decreased after the operation and recovered to normal levels within 3 years after the operation. This finding correlates with the clinical condition of bowel habits.

The resting pressure of the rectum elevated and remained high for more than 3 years in patients with rectal myectomy. This finding can be explained by the high tonus of the rectum oral to the aganglionic bowel which was left after rectal myectomy. The resting pressure of the rectum in patients treated by the PTCF method elevated just after the operation. It was lowered, however, to the normal level within about 3 years after the operation.

Regarding the data of basal rhythmic waves, no significant change was observed in comparison with normal controls.

The rectoanal reflex was observed only twice out of the 42 studies in patients with rectal myectomy and in nine of 137 studies in patients treated by the PTCF method. There was no relationship between the presence of reflex and clinical bowel habits.

Zusammenfassung

Anorektale manometrische Untersuchungen wurden 42mal bei 13 Patienten nach rektaler Myektomie und 137mal bei 49 Patienten nach „posterior triangular colonic flap" (PTCF) durchgeführt.

Der Ruhedruck im Analkanal war unmittelbar postoperativ erniedrigt und blieb unter den Werten gesunder Kontrollpatienten bei den Kindern mit rektaler Myektomie. Dies wurde auf die Resektion der Lamina muscularis im Analkanal zurückgeführt. Andererseits nahm der Ruhedruck bei Patienten mit PTCF nach der Operation ab und kehrte binnen 3 Jahren auf Normalwerte zurück. Diese Befunde stimmen mit den klinischen Beobachtungen des Stuhlverhaltens überein.

Der Ruhedruck im Rektum war erhöht und blieb hoch über mehr als 3 Jahre bei Patienten mit rektaler Myektomie. Dieser Befund wird erklärt durch den hohen Tonus des Rektums proximal des aganglionären Darmes, der bei der rektalen Myektomie zurückblieb. Der Ruhedruck im Rektum bei Patienten, die mit PTCF behandelt wurden, stieg unmittelbar nach der Operation an, erreichte jedoch 3 Monate nach der Operation wieder Normalwerte.

Hinsichtlich der rhythmischen Wellenbewegungen waren keine signifikanten Unterschiede zu den gesunden Kontrollen zu beobachten.

---

[1] Division of Pediatric Surgery, Tohoku University School of Medicine, 1-1, Seiryo-Machi, Sendai, 980 Japan
[2] Division of Pediatric Surgery, Tohoku University School of Medicine, Sendai, Japan

Ein rektoanaler Reflex wurde nur 2mal bei den 42 Untersuchungen der Patienten mit rektaler Myektomie gefunden und nur 9mal bei den 137 Untersuchungen der Patienten, die mit der PTCF-Methode behandelt wurden. Es fand sich kein Zusammenhang zwischen der Anwesenheit des Reflexes und dem klinischen Stuhlverhalten.

Résumé

Des examens par manométrie rectale ont été effectués 42 fois chez 13 patients après amputation rectale et 137 fois chez 49 patients après transposition colique (PTCF, posterior triangular colonic flap).
  La pression de repos dans le canal anal avait baissé immédiatement après l'opération et, dans le cas des enfants ayant subi une amputation rectale, elle resta en dessous des données obtenues chez des patients témoins. Cela fut imputé à la résection de la lamina muscularis dans le canal anal. D'autre part, la pression au repos chez les patients avec PTCF augmenta après l'opération et redevint normale en l'espace de 3 ans. Ces données confirment les observations cliniques de la fonction de défécation.
  La pression au repos dans le rectum a augmenté et est restée trop élevée pendant plus de 3 ans chez les patients ayant subi une amputation rectale. Cela s'explique par la tonicité élevée du rectum au niveau de l'intestin aganglionnaire, préservé par l'amputation rectale. La pression de repos dans le rectum chez les patients traités par PTCF augmenta immédiatement en post-opérative mais retrouva un niveau normal 3 mois après l'intervention.
  En ce qui concerne les ondulations rythmiques, aucune différence significative n'a été notée avec les témoins sains.
  Un réflexe recto-anal n'a été observé que 2 fois sur 42 examens de patients ayant subi une amputation rectale et 9 fois seulement sur les 137 examnes de patients traités selon la méthode PTCF. Il ne paraît y avoir aucun rapport entre la présence du réflexe et l'observation clinique de la défécation.

Introduction

There have been many investigations regarding the pathophysiology, diagnosis, and surgical treatment of patients with Hirschsprung's disease. In most reports the postoperative anorectal function was considered to be fair by the sporadic analyses according to clinical and manometrical bases (Holschneider et al. 1980; Suzuki et al. 1970; Frenckner and Lindstrom 1983). Several researchers (Suzuki et al. 1984; Nagasaki et al. 1980) reported the physiological changes of the anorectal function during their postoperative courses. We also investigated by serial manometric studies the results of physiological motility of the anorectum, mainly in patients having had rectal myectomy (Lynn 1966), and compared them with those of patients subjected to the posterior triangular colonic flap (PTCF) method (Kasai et al. 1977), which is modified Duhamel's procedure with complete internal sphincterotomy.

Materials

In the past 16 years, 30 cases of Hirschsprung's disease have been treated by rectal myectomy and 65 cases by the PTCF method at the Division of Pediatric Surgery,

Tohoku University Hospital. Anorectal manometric studies were performed 42 times on 13 out of the 30 patients undergoing rectal myectomy and 137 times on 48 out of the 60 cases treated by the PTCF method. Fourteen controls with normal bowel habits, ranging from neonates to adults, were included in the present study.

Methods

As a rule, anorectal manometry was performed preoperatively and about 1, 3, 6, and 12 months after the radical operation to clarify the physiological alteration in anorectal motility after the operation. Thereafter, the patients underwent manometric studies once or twice a year, but when the patients showed unsatisfactory bowel habits, the studies were repeated frequently. The results of the manometric studies are summarized into four categories according to the postoperative period, namely within 2 months, within 1 year, within 3 years, and over 3 years.

For manometry, the infusion open-tip method was employed. The pressure sensor (8 F in size and 90 cm in length) consisted of a polyethylene catheter with 1.2×2.0 mm side hole. Distilled water was infused at a rate of 0.82 ml/min using a Harvard pump (Model 975). The response was 35 mm Hg/s in the whole system. All data were recorded using a transducer (Gould P23ID) and polygraph system (amplifier, Nihon-Koden AP621G; recorder, Nihon-Koden WI 641G). After the catheter system was inserted into the anorectum, the anorectal resting pressure profile was first obtained by rapid withdrawal. Then, anorectal basal rhythmic waves were recorded using a resting pressure monitoring device. Finally, the rectoanal reflex in response to the distension of the rectum was examined.

The data of this study were analyzed by Student's t test, with significance being attributed to values of less than $P = 0.05$.

Results

Resting Pressure Profile

In the normal controls, as shown in Table 1 and Fig. 1, the length of the anal canal varied from about 1 cm in neonates to about 4 cm in adults. Although the resting pressure of the rectum remained unchanged (less than 10 mm Hg), the resting pressure of the anal canal elevated along with the length of the anal canal. A rectoanal reflex was present in all normal controls.

In patients with Hirschsprung's disease (Table 2), the resting pressure of the rectum and the anal canal and the length of the anal canal before surgery were 7.6 ± 2.7 mm Hg, 46.2 ± 25.5 mm Hg, and 2.3 ± 0.6 cm, respectively. These results were significantly different from those of normal infants. A rectoanal reflex was not detected in any patient. In patients after rectal myectomy the above measurements were performed within 2 months, 2–12 months, 1–3 years, and after 3 years

Table 1. Results of anorectal manometry in normal controls

	Resting pressure of rectum (mmHg)	Resting pressure of anal canal (mmHg)	Length of anal canal (cm)	Rectoanal reflex (%)
Neonates and infants ($n = 4$) (9 days–3 months)	4.8 ± 1.1	25.9 ± 9.2	1.1 ± 0.6	100
Younger children ($n = 4$) (1–3 years)	8.3 ± 0.6	38.2 ± 7.5	2.6 ± 0.7	100
Older children ($n = 4$) (6–10 years)	6.9 ± 0.2	63.0 ± 18.2	3.0 ± 0.7	100
Adults ($n = 4$) (>15 years)	8.2 ± 1.8	71.0 ± 10.1	4.1 ± 0.4	100

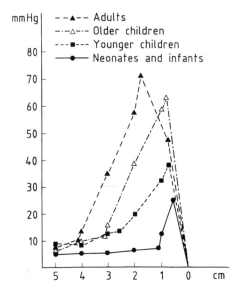

Fig. 1. Resting pressure profile of the anorectum in normal controls

Table 2. Results of anorectal manometry in patients with Hirschsprung's disease after rectal myectomy ($n = 13$)

Postoperative period	Resting pressure of rectum (mmHg)	Resting pressure of anal canal (mmHg)	Length of anal canal (cm)	Rectoanal reflex (%)
Before the operation	7.6 ± 2.7	46.2 ± 25.4	2.3 ± 0.6	0
Within 2 months	9.0 ± 2.0	32.8 ± 11.7	2.6 ± 0.5	0
2–12 months	7.8 ± 1.9	36.1 ± 18.9	2.6 ± 0.4	16.2
1–3 years	10.4 ± 3.0	34.2 ± 9.0	2.7 ± 1.0	12.5
More than 3 years	10.5 ± 4.6	38.3 ± 20.0	2.9 ± 0.6	0

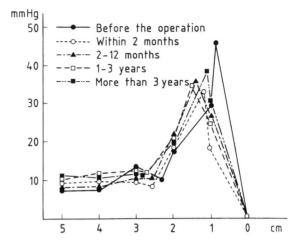

Fig. 2. Resting pressure profile of the anorectum in patients with rectal myectomy

Table 3. Results of anorectal manometry in patients with Hirschsprung's disease after PTCF treatment ($n = 49$)

Postoperative period	Resting pressure of rectum (mmHg)	Resting pressure of anal canal (mmHg)	Length of anal canal (cm)	Rectoanal reflex (%)
Before the operation	7.6 ± 2.7	46.2 ± 25.4	2.3 ± 0.6	0
Within 2 months	9.2 ± 3.9	32.2 ± 15.2	2.1 ± 0.4	0
2–12 months	8.7 ± 2.8	29.3 ± 12.6	2.1 ± 0.7	20
1–3 years	8.1 ± 3.0	35.4 ± 20.6	2.2 ± 0.8	7.4
More than 3 years	7.5 ± 3.7	51.7 ± 27.4	2.7 ± 0.7	8.3

(Table 2, Fig. 2). Although the difference was not statistically significant, the resting pressure of the rectum elevated immediately after the operation and remained high for more than 3 years. On the other hand, the resting pressure of the anal canal lowered moderately after myectomy (N.S.) and remained at levels lower than those of normal controls (N.S.). However, the differences between these results after the operation and those of age-matched controls were also not statistically significant. The anal canal showed a reasonable lengthening with physical growth.

The results of manometric studies in patients subjected to the PTCF method are shown in Table 3 and Fig. 3. The resting pressure of the rectum elevated right after the operation (N.S.) but lowered to normal levels within 3 years. The resting pressure of the anal canal which had decreased after operation (N.S.) also recovered to the normal level within 3 years. The differences between the postoperative data on patients and those on age-matched controls were not statistically significant.

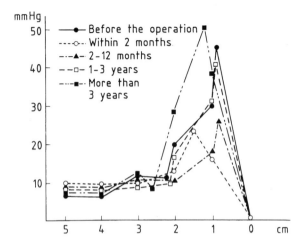

Fig. 3. Resting pressure profile of the anorectum in patients with PTCF method

The length of the anal canal shortened slightly (N.S.) but attained that in controls within 3 years.

Basal Rhythmic Waves

In normal controls, although the basal rhythmic waves of the rectum decreased in number with age, those of the anal canal remained almost unchanged (Table 4). Before operation in patients with Hirschsprung's disease (Table 5), the basal rhythmic waves of the rectum and the anal canal were 40.0 ± 14.7 and 12.7 ± 10.1 counts per minute, respectively; these levels were not statistically different from those of normal infants.

As illustrated in Table 5, the basal rhythmic waves in the two groups of patients after corrective surgery demonstrated a similar alteration in the course of few years. Just after the operation, the number of rhythmic waves of the rectum decreased (N.S.), and that of the anal canal increased (N.S.). However, these changes adjusted to normal levels within a few years after the radical operation.

Table 4. Basal rhythmic waves in normal controls (counts/min)

	Rectum	Anal canal
Neonates and infants ($n = 4$) (9 days–3 months)	40.1 ± 11.7	12.1 ± 3.2
Younger children ($n = 4$) (1–3 years)	28.2 ± 5.4	13.6 ± 2.4
Older children ($n = 3$) (6–10 years)	27.3 ± 4.2	13.0 ± 3.1
Adults ($n = 3$) (>15 years)	25.3 ± 4.1	13.4 ± 2.7

Table 5. Basal rhythmic waves after rectal myectomy and PTCF (counts/min)

Postoperative period	Rectal myectomy (n = 13)		PTCF (n = 49)	
	Rectum	Anal canal	Rectum	Anal canal
Before the operation	40.0 ± 14.7	12.7 ± 10.1	40.0 ± 14.7	12.7 ± 10.1
Within 2 months	34.7 ± 8.9	21.2 ± 11.4	31.8 ± 6.9	14.5 ± 6.6
2–12 months	31.1 ± 8.5	13.1 ± 2.3	35.2 ± 9.6	19.3 ± 13.5
1–3 years	36.3 ± 12.0	11.4 ± 1.9	30.0 ± 11.5	14.3 ± 4.8
More than 3 years	27.5 ± 5.4	12.4 ± 2.2	27.9 ± 8.8	12.4 ± 2.6

Rectoanal Reflex in Patients After Corrective Surgery

The rectoanal reflex was observed only twice during the 42 examinations of patients having had rectal myectomy. The rectoanal reflex was also observed in nine of 137 studies in patients treated by the PTCF method. The relationship between positive reflex and age is shown in Tables 2 and 3.

Discussion

Physiologically, Hirschsprung's disease retains an aspect of anal achalasia, that is, the long anal canal has a high resting pressure and an absence of the normal rectoanal reflex. The anal achalasia is released and the resting pressure of the anal canal rapidly lowered when the internal sphincter is divided, and the normal bowel is anastomosed. However, within 3 years the resting pressure of the anal canal recovers with the development of the surrounding muscle components as the patient grows. This subjective finding correlates well with the fact that the majority of postoperative patients with this disease obtain a satisfactory bowel habit within 3 years. We observed that the recovery of the resting pressure of the anal canal was delayed in patients with rectal myectomy compared to those treated by the PTCF method. Strip-shaped complete excision of the muscle layer of the internal sphincter causes this phenomenon. According to the report of Nagasaki and coworkers (1980), the resting pressure of the anal canal in patients treated by the Duhamel-Ikeda method gradually decreases and reaches normal levels.

The resting pressure of the rectum in patients treated by the PTCF method elevated temporarily, probably because of straining of the bowel by the operative maneuver. Thereafter, it lowered to normal levels by the releasing of the strain, along with the favorable bowel movement. On the other hand, the resting pressure of the rectum in patients with rectal myectomy gradually increased. Although the anal achalasia was relieved by rectal myectomy, an aganglionic bowel was left as it was. The normal bowel oral to the aganglionic bowel must increase the tension to propulse the intestinal content through the distal aganglionic bowel (Hashimoto et al. 1982). The resting pressure of the rectum after this procedure resulted in the high levels.

Some authors have reported that the basal rhythmic waves of the anal canal decreased after the operation (Tsukamoto 1985; Hirai 1984), but others have reported results similar to ours (Nagasaki 1979). Although the waves of the rectum decreased in the course of the postoperative priod in our studies, this may be attributed to aging. We think that the slight changes in basal rhythmic waves in patients after the corrective operations has no significance for the anorectal function.

There have been many reports (Holschneider et al. 1980; Nagasaki et al. 1980; Tsukamoto 1985; Hirai 1984; Nagasaki 1979; Shermeta and Nilprabhassorn 1977) concerning the rectoanal reflex after the surgical treatment of Hirschsprung's disease. Most of these emphasize that the rectoanal reflex is frequently observed in patients showing a favorable anorectal function. However, we found substantial differences in incidence according to the procedures employed. We were not able to observe the reflex frequently even in the patients with satisfactory bowel habits, either in those receiving rectal myectomy or in those receiving the PTCF method. We think that the presence of the reflex after the operation for Hirschsprung's disease does not have much significance for the clinical anorectal function. Recently, Suzuki et al. (1979) and Kunieda et al. (1985) observed that the aganglionic rectum has no motility, but the motility of the ganglionic bowel, pulled-through and anastomosed to the rectum, was demonstrated radiologically and endoscopically. The rectoanal reflex should originate mainly in the ganglionic bowel at the site of the anal canal.

References

Frenckner B, Lindstrom O (1983) Ano-rectal function assessed by manometry and electromyography after endorectal pull-through for Hirschsprung's disease. Z Kinderchir 38:101–104

Hashimoto K, Iwai N, Ogita S, et al (1982) Results of Hirschsprung's disease. J Jpn Soc Pediatr Surg 18:1029–1033 (in Japanese)

Hirai H (1984) Assessment of fecal continence with anorectal manometry after two different surgical procedures for Hirschsprung's disease. J Jpn Soc Pediatr Surg 20:1135–1147 (in Japanese)

Holschneider AM, Boerner W, Buurman O, et al (1980) Clinical and electromanometrical investigations of postoperative continence in Hirschsprung's disease. An international workshop. Z Kinderchir 29:39–48

Kasai M, Suzuki H, Ohi R, et al (1977) Rectoplasty with posterior triangular colonic flap – a radical new operation for Hirschsprung's disease. J Pediatr Surg 12:207–211

Kunieda K, Ohnishi A, Kunii Y, et al (1985) Anorectal manometry by electric stimulation under endoscopic observation. J Jpn Soc Pediatr Surg 21:336 (in Japanese)

Lynn HB (1966) Rectal myectomy for aganglionic megacolon. Mayo Clin Proc 41:289–295

Nagasaki A (1979) Manometric and radiologic study on anal continence in children with Hirschsprung's disease. J Jpn Soc Pediatr Surg 15:13–40 (in Japanese)

Nagasaki A, Ikeda K, Suita S (1980) Postoperative sequential anorectal manometric study of children with Hirschsprung's disease. J Pediatr Surg 15:615–619

Shermeta DW, Nilprabhassorn P (1977) Posterior myectomy for primary and secondary short segment aganglionosis. Am J Surg 133:39–41

Suzuki H, Watanabe K, Kasai M (1970) Manometric and cineradiographic studies on anorectal motility in Hirschsprung's disease before and after surgical operation. Tohoku J exp Med 192:69–80

Suzuki H, Tsukamoto Y, Amano S, et al (1984) Motility of the anorectum after "rectoplasty with posterior triangular colonic flap" in Hirschsprung's disease. Jpn J Surg 14:335–338

Suzuki H, Yamashita T, Saijo H, et al (1979) Motility of the intestine after Martin's procedure. J Jpn Soc Pediatr Surg 15:775–777 (in Japanese)

Tsukamoto Y (1985) Manometric studies on motility of the ano-rectum after rectoplasty with posterior triangular colonic flap for Hirschsprung's disease. J Jpn Soc Pediatr Surg 21:645–658 (in Japanese)

Continence and Reflex Pressure Profile After Surgery to Correct the Imperforate Anus

M. Ishihara and K. Morita

Summary

To clarify the cause of constipation which follows surgery for the supralevator type of disorder associated with the imperforate anus, rectal compliance, percentage maximum static anorectal pressure, and reflex profile were measured by anorectal manometry in 108 normal controls and 42 patients. Patients with constipation had a low percentage anorectal pressure (50%), high rectal compliance, associated with megarectum, and defecation of the staining type with constipation due to a reaction in anorectal motility.

Zusammenfassung

Um die Ursache der Obstipation nach Operation einer supralevatorischen Analatresie aufzudecken, wurden Messungen der rektalen Compliance, des maximalen statischen anorektalen Druckes (in %) und des Reflexprofiles bei 42 Patienten und 108 gesunden Kontrollen durchgeführt. Patienten mit Obstipation hatten einen niedrigen anorektalen Druck (50%) und eine hohe rektale Compliance, die mit einem Megarektum und Obstipation mit Überlaufenkopresis aufgrund der veränderten anorektalen Motilität verbunden waren.

Résumé

Afin de connaître l'étiologie d'une constipation après opération pour atrésie anale supralévatoire, on a procédé à des mesures de la compliance rectale, de la pression maximale statique anorectale (en %) et de la présence de réflexes dans le cas de 42 patients et de 108 témoins sains. Chez les patients présentant une constipation, la pression anorectale était basse (50%) et la compliance rectale élevée, cette dernière étant liée à un megarectum et à une constipation avec spotting dus à la modification de la motilité anorectale.

Introduction

After surgery to correct the imperforate anus, 80%–90% of patients whose disorder was of the translevator type had good continence, but of patients treated for the supralevator type of condition, only 20%–50% had good continence (Tailor and Zachary 1973; Iwai et al. 1979; Ito et al. 1981; Nagasaki et al. 1983). Incontinence and constipation are part of the pattern of abnormal defecation which oc-

First Department of Surgery, Nihon University School of Medicine, 30 Ooyaguchi-Kamimachi, Itabsai-ku, Tokyo 173, Japan

curs in patients with the supralevator type of disorders. Causes of the incontinence which follows surgery for the supralevator type of disorders were examined by objective assessments, which were made by various radiological techniques (Cywes et al. 1971; Kelly 1972), computed tomography (Ikawa et al. 1985), anorectal manometry (Schärli and Kiesewetter 1969; Schnaufer et al. 1967; Ahran et al. 1976; Iwai et al. 1979; Nagasaki et al. 1983), and electromyography (Tailor and Zachary 1973; Ito et al. 1981). These studies revealed causes of incontinence which were due to the failure to utilize the external and puborectal muscles at surgery. By contrast, the factors responsible for constipation remain to be elucidated. The purpose of this study was to determine some of the factors which cause constipation after surgery for the supralevator type of disorders.

Patients and Methods

A total of 108 normal controls and 42 patients who had undergone surgery for imperforate anus between 1962 and 1981 at the First Department of Surgery, Nihon University School of Medicine were studied. Normal subject (42 women, 66 men) ranged in age from 3 days to 70 years. The measurement of percent maximum static anorectal pressure was performed with all controls, and the reflex pressure profiles and tests of rectal compliance were made with 29 controls (12 girls, 17 boys) who ranged in age from 5 to 20 years (mean, 10.0 ± 5.5 years). Assessment of continence was based on the following criteria: (a) normal defecation, with normal spontaneous bowel movements without soiling or with infrequent soiling; (b) constipation, defined here as persistent constipation relieved only by irrigation of the bowel or laxatives, with only occasional soiling; (c) incontinence, defined in the same way as constipation, but with soiling despite irrigations, or complete incontinence. The 42 patients (4 girls, 38 boys) were from 5 to 20 years old (mean, 10.0 ± 5.5 years).

Table 1 shows the type of disorder and the surgical methods used. All patients who had a translevator type of disorder were treated by the perineal approach. Of the patients who had disorders to the supralevator type, 14 were treated by the new abdominoperineal approach, in which the puborectal muscle is exposed directly

Table 1. Types of disorder and surgical procedures

Type of disorder	Number of patients	Surgical procedure				
		PA	APA (new)	APA (old)	SAP	Secondary
Translevator	9	9				
Supralevator	33		14	6	3	10

PA, Perineal anoplasty; APA (new), new method of abdominoperineal anoplasty; APA (old), old method of abdominoperineal anoplasty; SAP, sacro-abdominoperineal anoplasty; Secondary, patient had undergone surgery initially at another hospital

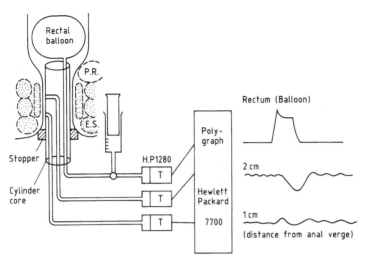

Fig. 1. Schematic representation of the system for anorectal manometric studies. Two open-tipped catheters within a cylindrical core were placed 4 cm and 3 cm from the anal verge and then withdrawn 2 cm to a position 2 cm and 1 cm from the verge, respectively. The whole apparatus was held against the perianal skin during the test by a cylindrical bored stopper. *P.R.*, Puborectal muscle; *E.S.*, external muscle; *T.*, Transducer

in the pelvis by pushing up the perineal wound with the forefinger slowly and carefully toward the pelvis. Six patients with the supralevator type of disorder were treated by the old abdominoperineal approach, which does not pay particular attention to the puborectal muscle. Three patients were treated by a sacro-abdominoperineal approach. Ten patients had undergone surgery on the anal area at another hospital. All children were examined without special preparation of the bowel, except those patients who had fecal masses removed by repeated enemas. A sedative (monosodium trichlorethyl phosphate, 100–150 mg/kg) was given only to those patients aged 4 years or younger.

First, the static pressure in the anal canal was measured with a 50-cm polyethylene tube (internal diameter, 1 mm) with a side hole. The catheter was connected to a transducer (YHP 1280c) and to a polygraph (YHP 7700, Hewlett Packared, USA). Distilled water was infused at a constant rate of 1 ml/min, produced by nitrogen gas pressure and an Arndorfer's internal pressure (Arndorfer et al. 1977) measurement system (SN 632, Star Medical Japan). The station pull-through method was used, and the measurements were made in the anorectum, 1–5 cm from the anal verge. The values obtained from 42 patients after surgery to correct an imperforate anus were expressed as a percentage of the analogous values obtained from 108 age-matched controls.

The next measurements were those of the rectoanal reflex. The apparatus used in the present study was specially designed for testing and recording the pressure of the anal canal in children (Fig. 1). The probe was basically an open-tipped system, consisting of a cylindrical core in which two polyethylene tubes, each 1 mm in diameter, were attached to the core, 1 cm apart. A latex balloon was also attached to the polyethylene tube and was connected, through the core, to a syringe by a three-way stopcock set for flexible distension of the rectum. The three open-tipped tubes, two for measuring the pressure in the anal canal and one for the balloon system, were connected to the transducer. The probe was passed through the anal canal so that balloon lay in the distal rectum, and the orifices of the open-tipped tubes were lodged 4 cm and 3 cm from the anal verge, respectively, for the first part of the test. The apparatus was then withdrawn 2 cm, so that the tubes became fixed 2 cm and 1 cm, respectively, from the anal verge (see Fig. 1). After the recording system was operated for 15 min, the anorectal-sphincteric response to distension of the balloon was recorded directly on the tracing. Our protocol for rectal stimuli consisted of injecting 10–100 ml air into the balloon in 5 s and maintaining the resultant state of inflation for 10 s. This procedure began with a minimal volume and was continued until more than the critical volume was reached, with intervals of 1 mm between each distension.

The pressure-volume curve of the rectum was made by inflating the rectal balloon with different amounts of air and measuring the corresponding pressure in the balloon. Rectal compliance was calculated by dividing the changes in volume (ml) by the changes in pressure (mm Hg) on the linear portion of the curve. Rectal compliance is related to megarectum; therefore, we assessed the relationship between rectal compliance and the existence of megarectum using barium enemas.

Data were expressed as means ± SD, and statistical analyses were performed using Student's t-test. Values of less than $P = 0.05$ were considered to be significant.

Results

Nature of Original Anal Disorder and Subsequent Pattern of Defecation

Table 2 shows that all nine patients who had the translevator type of disorder had a normal pattern of defecation. Of the 33 patients who had the supralevator type of disorder, normal defecation was observed in 11, constipation in 10, and incontinence in 12.

Table 2. Types of disorder and subsequent pattern of defecation

Type of disorder	Number of patients	Number of controls	Pattern of defecation	
			Constipation	Incontinence
Translevator	9	9		
Supralevator	33	11	10	12

Percentage of Maximum Static Pressure in the Anal Canal

Table 3 shows the maximum pressure in the anal canal, as measured in 108 controls. Grouped by age, the pressure was 20.3 ± 6.6 mmHg in 25 subjects 3 weeks older or younger, 30.5 ± 5.9 mmHg in 35 subjects aged 4 weeks–2 years, 44.0 ± 11.0 mmHg in 29 subjects aged 3–15 years, and 64.7 ± 17.2 mmHg in 19 subjects aged 16–70 years. Significant differences in the mean pressures were observed among these groups ($P < 0.01$). Table 4 shows the maximum values for static pressure in the anal canal for each type of disorder and pattern of defecation. The mean pressure was 24.5 mmHg in the nine patients who had a translevator type of disorder and abnormal defecation, but less than 20 mmHg in those who had a supralevator type of disorder. Those patients who had a normal pattern of defecation or were constipated showed higher values than those who were incontinent. The percentage maximum static pressure was calculated from the values of maximum static pressure of the patients and the controls. The mean percentage maximum static pressure was 55% in the patients who had a translevator type of disorder with normal defecation, and less than 50% in those who had a supralevator type of disorder. Those patients with incontinence had a mean value of less than 30%. Significant differences in these parameters were observed between the patients who had translevator types of disorders, those who had supralevator types of disorders with normal defecation or constipation, and those who had supralevator types of disorders with incontinence ($P < 0.01$–0.02).

Table 3. Mean static pressure in the anal canal in various age groups of normal subjects

Age group	Number of patients	Mean static pressure (mmHg)
Under 3 weeks	25	20.3 ± 6.6
4 weeks–2 years	35	30.5 ± 5.9
3–15 years	29	44.0 ± 11.0
16–70 years	18	64.7 ± 17.2

Significant differences were noted in the pressure among these groups

Table 4. Maximum static pressure and percentage maximum static pressure in patients after surgery for imperforate anus

Type of disorder	Pattern of defecation	Number of patients	Maximum static pressure (mmHg)	Percentage maximum static pressure
Translevator	Normal	9	24.5 ± 4.5	55.0 ± 15.3
Supralevator	Normal	11	16.7 ± 4.5	38.6 ± 8.3
	Constipation	10	18.9 ± 5.1	43.2 ± 12.3
	Incontinence	12	11.9 ± 4.8	27.4 ± 9.8

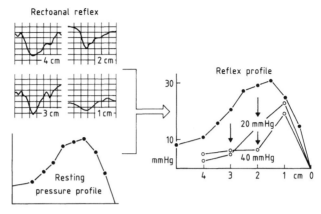

Fig. 2. Reflex anorectal pressure profile (reflex profile) in normal subjects, demonstrating active motility of the anorectum when the rectal pressure rises. Distances represent distance in cm centimeters anal verge

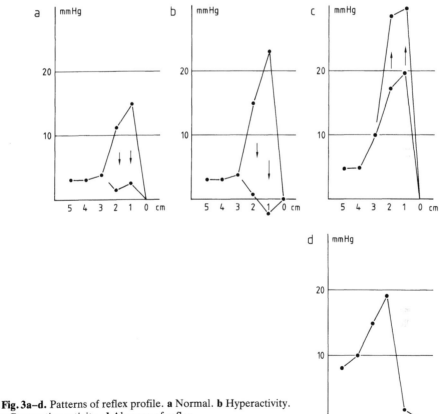

Fig. 3a–d. Patterns of reflex profile. **a** Normal. **b** Hyperactivity. **c** Contractive activity. **d** Absence of reflex

Profile of Reflex Anorectal Pressure

To assess active anorectal motility, as opposed to resting anorectal tonus, Hiramoto et al. (Hiramoto and Morita 1978) measured the profile of reflex anorectal pressure (reflex profile) by projecting the drop in pressure in response to rectal distension onto the profile of static anorectal pressure. In normal controls (5–20 years of age), it was demonstrated that the anorectum lost its tone from the upper functional anal canal by about 50%. The lower rectal pressure was 20 mm Hg, but by the last 1 cm of the anal canal, the rectal pressure could rise to 40 mm Hg (Fig. 2). Patients who had surgery for an imperforate anus showed four types of reflex profile, as illustrated in Fig. 3. Hyperactivity of relaxation was seen as increased contraction 1–2 cm from the anal verge. A contractive pattern of activity consisted of a contractive reflex 1–2 cm from the anal verge. The absence of reflex did not show any reflex activity in the anal canal. Table 5 shows the relationship between patterns of defecation and the four different reflex profiles. A normal pattern was observed in nine patients who had a translevator type of disorder. In the 11 patients who had a normal pattern of defecation and a supralevator type of disorders, three had a normal reflex profile, six demonstrated hyperactivity, one had a contractive profile, and one had no reflex profile. Of 12 incontinent patients, three had a contractive reflex profile and eight had no reflex profile.

Pressure-Volume Curves and Rectal Compliance

Pressure-volume curves (Fig. 4) for the patients with normal patterns of defecation and translevator and supralevator types of disorders were almost the same as the durve for normal controls. The curve for the patients who had constipation with the supralevator type of disorder was flatter, and that of patients who were incontinent with the supralevator type of disorder was steeper than those of normal subjects. Table 6 shows that in patients with the translevator type of disorder, 11 patients with normal patterns of defecation had normal rectum, and only two patients had a megarectum. Rectal compliance of seven patients without megarectum was similar to that of the normal controls. In patients with the supralevator type of disorder, 10 of 11 patients with normal defecation had a normal

Table 5. Patterns of reflex profile

Type of disorder	Pattern of defecation	Number of patients	Pattern of reflex profile			
			Normal	Hyperactivity	Contraction	Absence
Translevator	Normal	9	9			
Supralevator	Normal	11	3	6	1	1
	Constipation	10	2	2	5	1
	Incontinence	12	1		3	8

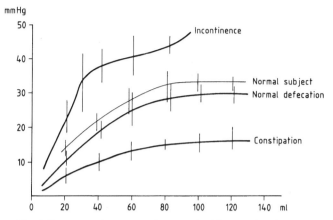

Fig. 4. Pressure-volume curve in normal subjects and patients

Table 6. Rectal compliance

Subjects or type of disorder	Pattern of defecation	With or without megarectum	Number of patients	Rectal compliance (ml/mm Hg)
Normal control			29	2.45 ± 1.5
Translevator type	Normal defecation	Without	7	2.20 ± 0.66
		With	2	3.99 ± 2.4
Supralevator type	Normal defecation	Without	10	2.17 ± 0.75
		With	1	3.5
	Constipation	With	9	4.58 ± 1.44
		Without	1	2.0
	Incontinence	Without	12	1.42 ± 0.49

rectum and only one had megarectum. Nine of the ten patients who had constipation had megarectum, and only one had a normal rectum; 11 of 12 patients who were incontinent had a normal rectum. Rectal compliance with constipation was remarkably high, and that with incontinence was low. The difference was statistically significant between normal controls or patients with normal defecation without megarectum and patients with constipation with megarectum ($P < 0.01$), and between patients with constipation with megarectum and those with incontinence ($P < 0.02$).

Discussion

Postoperatively, many patients who have undergone surgical treatment for a supralevator type of disorder have abnormal patterns of defecation, such as incontinence and constipation. Patients with a translevator type of disorder are less prone to such problems. Several groups of researchers have attempted to measure factors involved in abnormal continence to make an objective assessment. Cywes et al. (1971) and Kelly (1972) developed various radiological techniques to investigate these factors; Ikawa et al. (1985) used computed tomography; Schärli and Kiesewetter (1969) used measurements of anorectosigmoid pressure; Schnaufer et al. (1967), Ahran et al. (1976), Iwai et al. (1979), and Nagasaki et al. (1983) examined the relationship between anal-canal pressure and the rectosphincteric reflex; and Tailor and Zachary (1973) and Ito et al. (1981) utilized the electromyography of the anal canal. These studies together demonstrated those factors involved in incontinence which were due to abnormal function of the anorectal structures, especially of the external sphincter and puborectal muscle. A variety of surgical procedures have been designed to permit adequate utilization of the external sphincter and puborectal muscle.

Some patients who had a supralevator type of disorder had constipation, no natural defecation without the use of enemas, and no soilings. The factors causing such constipation are still unknown. In the past, the postoperative clinical evaluation of patients with imperforate anus commonly utilized Kelly's score (Kelly 1972), which is based on three parameters: continence, staining, and sphincter squeezing. The last of these is used only to evaluate incontinence without constipation. Some factors involved in constipation in postoperative patients who had supralevator types of disorders were studied by anorectal manometry. For clinical evaluation, we used three parameters.

The measurement of static pressure in the anal canal is considered to be a simple and relatively objective method. However, values obtained from different institutions cannot be compared directly because of the differences in techniques and conditions. For example, the normal value reported by Duthie and Watts (1965) was 40 mmHg for subjects aged 20–50 years, and that reported by Iwai et al. (1979) was 23.4 ± 1.9 cm H_2O. We used the value of the percentage maximum static pressure to evaluate the data obtained in different institutions. To calculate such values accurately, the normal control values must be known for each institution. The percentage maximum static pressure was 50% or more in those patients who had a translevator type of disorder with normal defecation, 30%–50% in those with a supralevator type of disorder and normal defecation or constipation, and 30% or lower in those who had a supralevator type of disorder with incontinence.

The rectosphincteric reflex test measures only the presence or absence of reflex at a point 2 cm from the anal verge. On the other hand, the reflex profile measures the rectosphincteric reflex at four points in the anal canal and is combined with the profile of static pressure in the anal canal. Thus, this test can be used to assess active anorectal motility. Postoperative patients with imperforate anus showed four types of reflex profile: normal, excessive relaxation, contraction, and absence of a reflex profile. All patients who had the translevator type of disorder had a normal reflex profile, 6 of 11 patients who had normal defecation with the supralevator type of disorder had profile indicative of excessive relaxation, and 3 of 11 had a normal reflex profile. On the other hand, 5 of 10 patients who had constipation had a contractive reflex profile, and 8 of 12 patients who were incontinent had a nonreactive reflex profile. The contractive reflex profile is considered to be caused by the contraction of the external muscle or the puborectal muscle. Rutter and Riddel (1975) examined electromyographically the puborectal muscle and anal pressure in patients who suffered from solitary ulcer syndrome of the rectum and constipation of the straining type. These patients showed the characteristic hyperactivity of the puborectal muscle. Therefore, we may assume that the patients who had constipation after treatment for the supralevator type of disorder had a pattern of constipation similar to the straining type.

Eisner (1972) and Suzuki et al. (1980) examined the relationship between rectal compliance in constipated patients with megacolon and found abnormally high rectal compliance in constipated children with megarectum. Eisner also reported that patients with incontinence after surgery to correct an imperforate anus had low rectal compliance. It appears, from their results and ours, that one of the factors in constipation after surgery for an imperforate anus is high rectal compliance associated with megarectum, and one of the factors in incontinence is low rectal compliance associated with impaired distensibility of the rectal wall.

Our conclusions are as follows:

1. The percentage maximum static pressure after surgery was 50% or less than that of normal controls and was not related to the pattern of the defecation.
2. Patients with normal patterns of defecation had lower pressure in the anal canal than normal controls but had normal or hyperrelaxed anorectal motility and normal distensibility of the rectal wall. In these patients, the interactions of anal-canal pressure, distensibility of the rectal wall, and anorectal motility were well balanced.
3. Patients with constipation had a reaction in anorectal motility and high rectal compliance, associated with megarectum. The stool remained in the rectum and was disturbed by the reaction in anorectal motility; this was sometimes associated with defecation of the staining type.
4. Patients with incontinence had low anal-canal pressure, an absence of anorectal motility, and low rectal compliance. All of these factors are related to incontinence. Kottmeier's repair (Kottmeier and Dziadiw 1967) or Pena's posterior sagittal repair (Pena 1986) are the treatments of choice for low pressure in the anal canal and absence of anorectal motility.

References

Ahran P, Faverdin C, Dubois F, Coupris L, Denys P (1976) Manometric assessment of continence after surgery for imperforate anus. J Pediatr Surg 11:157–166

Arndorfer RC, Stef JJ, Dodds W, Linehan JH, Hogan WJ (1977) Improved infusion system for intraluminal esophageal manometry. Gastroenterology 73:23–27

Cywes S, Cremin BJ, Low JH (1971) Assessment of continence after treatment for anorectal agenesis: a clinical and radiologic correlation. J Pediatr Surg 6:132–137

Duthie HL, Watts JM (1965) Contribution of the external anal sphincter to the pressure zone in the anal canal. Gut 6:64–68

Eisner M (1972) Function examination of rectum and anus in normals, in disturbances of continence and defecation, and in congenital malformations. Scand J Gastroenterol 7:305–308

Hiramoto Y, Morita K (1978) Evaluation of surgical treatment of Hirschsprung's disease with reference to manometric studies. Nihon Univ J Med 20:307–317

Ikawa H, Yokoyama J, Sanbonmatu T, Hagane K, Endo M, Katumata K, Kohda E (1985) The use of computerized tomography to evaluate anorectal anomalies. J Pediatr Surg 20:640–644

Ito Y, Yokoyama J, Hayashi A, Ihara N, Katumata K (1981) Reappraisal of endorectal pull-through procedure. I. Anorectal malformations. J Pediatr Surg 16:476–483

Iwai N, Ogita S, Kida M, Fujita Y, Majima S (1979) A clinical and manometric correlation for assessment of postoperative continence in imperforate anus. J Pediatr Surg 14:538–543

Kelly JH (1972) The clinical and radiological assessment of anal continence in childhood. Aust NZ J Surg 42:62–63

Kottmeier PK, Dziadiw R (1967) The complete relese of the levator ani sling in fecal incontinence. J Pediatr Surg 2:111–117

Nagasaki A, Ikeda K, Hayasida Y, Sumitomo K, Samezima S (1983) Assessment of bowel control with anorectal manometry after surgery for anorectal malformation. Jpn J Surg 14:229–234

Pena A (1986) Posterior sagittal approach for the correction of anorectal malformation. Adv Surg 19:69–100

Rutter KRP, Riddel RH (1975) The solitary ulcer syndrome of the rectum. Clin Gastroenterol 4:505–530

Schärli AF, Kiesewetter WB (1969) Imperforate anus: anorectosigmoid pressure studies as a quantitative evaluation of postoperative continence. J Pediatr Surg 4:694–704

Schnaufer L, Talbert JL, Haller A, Tobon RF, Schuster MM (1967) Differential sphincter studies in the diagnosis of ano-rectal disorders of childhood. J Pediatr Surg 2:538–543

Suzuki H, Amano S, Honzumi M, Saizo H, Sakakura K (1980) Rectoanal pressure and rectal compliance in constipated infants and children. Z Kinderchir 4:330–336

Tailor HL, Zachary R (1973) Anal continence following surgery for imperforate anus. J Pediatr Surg 8:497–503

Management of Defecation in Spina Bifida

M. Maie, M. Sakaniwa, H. Takahashi, and J. Iwai

Summary

The main presenting complaint in defecational disorders in spina bifida is constipation. The principal cause of this complaint is hypofunction or paralysis of muscles in the pelvic floor as a result of the spinal cord injuries. To evaluate the present status of defecation, anorectal manometry with special reference to the anorectal pressure profile has been useful. The possibility of using anorectal manometry for the research of anorectal movement and participation of spinal cord was discussed.

Zusammenfassung

Die Obstipation steht bei den Defäkationsstörungen bei der Spina bifida im Vordergrund. Die Hauptursache dafür ist die Unterfunktion oder Lähmung der Beckenbodenmuskulatur aufgrund der Rückenmarkschädigung. Die anorektale Manometrie mit besonderer Berücksichtigung des anorektalen Druckprofils ist eine nützliche Methode zur Bestimmung des Ausmaßes der Defäkationsstörung. Die Möglichkeiten der anorektalen Manometrie bei der Erforschung der anorektalen Bewegungsabläufe und der Beteiligung des Rückenmarks werden diskutiert.

Résumé

La constipation constitue le trouble de la défécation le plus important dans les cas de spina bifida. La raison principale en est la diminution de la fonction ou la paralysie de la musculature du plancher pelvien dues à la lésion de la moëlle épinière. La manométrie anorectale et en particulier l'observation de la pression anorectale est une méthode d'une grande utilité dans la détermination de l'ampleur des troubles de la défécation. Les auteurs discutent des possibilités offertes par la manométrie pour l'étude de la motilité anorectale et la participation éventuelle de la moëlle épinière.

Introduction

With recognition of the effectiveness of early closure in spina bifida, especially in open myelomeningocele, significant improvements have been made in the treatment of hydrocephalus, motor disturbances of the lower limbs, and micturitional disturbances (Lorber 1971). However, the pathophysiology and treatment of defecational problems due to the same causes as micturitional disturbances and lower

Department of Pediatric Surgery, Chiba University 1-8-1, Inohana, Chiba, Japan limb deformities unfortunately have not been considered as important in achieving a better quality of life for patients with these problems (White and Shaker 1974).

The cause of defecational disturbance is malfunction of the terminal colon due mainly to neuronal lesion. Constipation and fecal mass retention with eventual dilatation of the terminal colon and rectum are symptomatic consequences. Before infants take solid food, their stool is generally soft and easy to evacuate by manual manipulation, such as by Credé's maneuver, with simultaneous bladder expression. We have therefore introduced this technique in early infancy to control fecal and urinal disorders.

The aim of this work is to analyze the results of these managements on defecational problems.

Patients and Methods

During the past 20 years we have had treated 87 cases of open spina bifida and 72 cases of closed spina bifida. To be certain as to the nature of their problems with defecation, we selected a series patients with spina bifida over 3 years; of these 33 cases were of open spina bifida and 28 of closed spina bifida.

Patients were classified into four groups according to the urgency of treatment by means of enemas or suppositories to evacuate fecal mass. These groups were: (a) normal, no particular treatment necessary; (b) good, almost no treatment necessary; (c) fair, particular treatment necessary about once a week; and (d) poor, continuous treatment necessary.

As a subjective evaluation of bowel function, anorectal manometry was used. Among the data obtained in this investigation, the pressure profile of the anal canal and the anorectal inhibitory reflex were used to analyze bowel function. The pressure profile was divided into three groups (Fig. 1): (a) normal, identical to

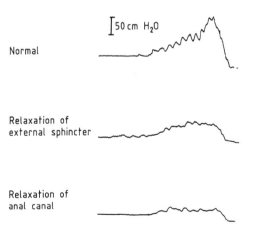

Fig. 1. Patterns of the anorectal pressure profile in spina bifida

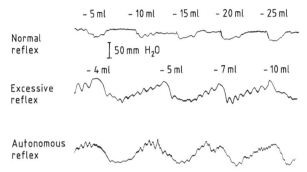

Fig. 2. Patterns of the anorectal inhibitory reflex in spina bifida

normal subjects, a high-pressure zone occurred in the anal-canal pressure profile; (b) relaxation of external sphincter, the high-pressure zone disappeared, and the internal sphincter wave form was predominant throughout the anal canal; and (c) relaxation of anal canal, pressure rise was almost nil throughout the anal canal.

The rectoanal inhibitory reflex (RIR) was used to divide subjects into three groups according to the reaction to rectal distension (Fig. 2): (a) normal reflex, normal RIR was present; (b) excessive reflex, the basic rhythmical wave was high, and RIR was accelerated with minimal distention; and (c) autonomous reflex, wave form similar to RIR was present even without any rectal distention.

Results

Clinical Assessment of Defecation. In the open spina bifida patients, there were no instances of the normal type, and 16 cases were classified as good, 15 cases as fair, and 2 cases as poor. In the cases of closed spina bifida, the normal type was found in 10, the good in 5, the fair in 10, and the poor in only 3 cases (Table 1). This dis-

Table 1. Clinical assessment of defecation in spina bifida

Type of spina bifida	Maximal height of lesion	Clinical assessment of defecation			
		Normal	Good	Fair	Poor
Open		0	16	15	2
	Thorax	0	2	0	0
	Lumbar	0	11	10	0
	Sacral	0	3	5	2
Closed		10	5	10	3
	Thorax	0	0	0	1
	Lumbar	5	1	4	2
	Sacral	5	4	6	0

tribution suggests that even in open spina bifida, if the appropriate maneuver is undertaken to evacuate fecal mass in early infancy, a good control of defecation can be achieved. But care must be taken regarding defecation even in closed spina bifida because more than half of our patients needed some other treatment due to defecational disturbance.

Anorectal Manometry. In the 33 cases of open spina bifida, the external relaxation type was observed in 14 cases, and relaxation of anal canal was found in 9 (i.e., in a total of 71%). In the 28 cases of closed spina bifida, abnormal patterns were observed in 12 cases in each subtype (i.e., in a total of 43%: Table 2). Thus, there exist differences in the degree of paralysis of the external sphincter among these in each spina bifida group ($P < 0.05$, by Wilcoxon's ordered-rank test). The maximal anal pressure at rest in the patients of normal type was approximately the same as in normal subjects, and it decreased with the progression of anal-canal hypotonicity (Table 3). Comparing the clinical assessment and the anorectal pressure profile, it seems likely that advanced paralysis of the anal canal tends to worsen the clinical assessment (Table 4).

Table 2. Patterns of anorectal pressure profile in spina bifida

Type of spina bifida	Maximal height of lesion	Anorectal pressure profile		
		Normal	Relaxation of external sphincter	Relaxation of anal canal
Open		10	14	9
	Thorax	0	1	1
	Lumbar	8	11	2
	Sacral	2	2	6
Closed		16	6	6
	Thorax	1	0	0
	Lumbar	9	1	2
	Sacral	6	5	4

Table 3. Maximal anal pressure (cm H_2O) and anorectal pressure profile in the spina bifida

Type of spina bifida	Anorectal pressure profile		
	Normal	Relaxation of external sphincter	Relaxation of anal canal
Open	94.5 ± 35.5 ($n = 10$)	55.4 ± 16.6 ($n = 14$)	36.5 ± 10.7 ($n = 9$)
Closed	91.1 ± 29.1 ($n = 16$)	57.1 ± 13.8 ($n = 6$)	25.4 ± 4.3 ($n = 6$)

Table 4. Clinical assessment of defecation and anorectal pressure profile in spina bifida

Anorectal pressure profile	Clinical assessment of defecation[a]			
	Normal	Good	Fair	Poor
Normal	9 (0)	8 (5)	9 (5)	0
Relaxation of external sphincter	1 (0)	9 (7)	8 (6)	2 (1)
Relaxation of anal canal	0	4 (4)	8 (4)	3 (1)

[a] Figures represent the numbers for both open and closed forms of spina bifida, those in parentheses specifically of the open form

Table 5. Type of spina bifida and rectoanal inhibitory reflex

Type of spina bifida	Maximal height of lesion	Rectoanal inhibitory reflex		
		Normal reflex	Excessive reflex	Autonomous reflex
Open		15	9	9
	Thorax	1	1	0
	Lumbar	10	6	7
	Sacral	4	2	2
Closed		19	6	3
	Thorax	0	1	0
	Lumbar	8	2	0
	Sacral	11	3	3

Rectoanal Inhibitory Reflex. All cases exhibited the RIR. The pathological reflex in spina bifida was characterized by the ease with which the reflex could be stimulated by rectal distention and by an excessive reflex with stimulation. This was the typical finding in patients of the normal type. In the open spina bifida group, normal reflex was present in 15 cases, excessive reflex in 9, and autonomous reflex in 9. In the closed spina bifida group, the distribution of these types was 19, 6, and 3 cases, respectively (Table 5). Whereas 45% of patients with open spina bifida were classified as being of the normal type, 69% of those with closed spina bifida were of the normal type ($P < 0.05$, by Wilcoxon's ordered-rank test). The autonomous reflex was predominant among those with open spina bifida. However, there was no clear relationship between RIR and clinical assessment, and clinical assessment was not necessarily worse among those with the autonomous reflex (Table 6). The maximal anal pressure in relation to the pressure profile and the type of reflex is summarized in Table 7. The maximal anal pressure among those with the autonomous reflex was significantly higher than among those with other types of reflexes.

Table 6. Clinical assessment of defecation and rectoanal inhibitory reflex in spina bifida

Rectoanal inhibitory reflex	Clinical assessment of defecation[a]			
	Normal	Good	Fair	Poor
Normal reflex	9 (0)	12 (9)	10 (5)	3 (1)
Excessive reflex	1 (0)	5 (4)	9 (5)	0
Autonomous reflex	0	4 (3)	6 (5)	2 (1)

[a] Figures represent the numbers for both open and closed forms of spina bifida, those in parentheses specifically of the open form

Table 7. Maximal anal pressure (cm H_2O) in relation to anorectal pressure profile and rectoanal inhibitory reflex

Anorectal pressure profile	Rectoanal inhibitory reflex		
	Normal reflex	Excessive reflex	Autonomous reflex
Normal	83.4 ± 25.5 ($n = 18$)	97.2 ± 36.6 ($n = 5$)	130.5 ± 21.4 ($n = 3$)
Relaxation of external sphincter	54.3 ± 20.0 ($n = 10$)	51.2 ± 6.2 ($n = 5$)	64.4 ± 7.7 ($n = 5$)
Relaxation of anal canal	31.9 ± 12.0 ($n = 6$)	29.4 ± 4.6 ($n = 5$)	39.2 ± 10.0 ($n = 4$)

Discussion

Preventing dilatation of the colon and rectum after having solid stool makes defecation easier and helps prevent fecal impaction of the colon. If adequate care is not taken to ensure satisfactory defecation, stools become harder by the time that patients reach infancy or school age. The result is a constipated constitution and overflow incontinence in the extreme (Forrest 1976; White and Shaker 1974). Similar cases were encountered in patients whose back lesions had been treated in a different hospital without subsequent treatment to ease fecal evacuation. However, those patients who had received primary care in the neonatal period at our Pediatric Surgical Department did not present these difficulties. This suggests that early defecational training is an essential prerequisite to improving the patient's quality of life (White and Shaker 1974).

It is clear that the clinical assessment of defecation varies according to the condition of spina bifida. In the open spina bifida group, none of the patients studied was capable of normal defecation. By contrast, however, ten patients (36%) with closed spina bifida were able to be considered normal. There is no evidence to suggest any correlation between clinical assessment and the maximal height of the spinal lesion. While two of the open spina bifida cases with thoracic lesion were assessed as good, the two closed spina bifida patients with sacral lesion were given a poor assessment in terms of their defecational ability (see Table 1).

Analysis of different components of the anorectal pressure profile indicates that the slow wave in the oral side of the anal canal indicates the activity of the internal sphincter. The high-pressure zone on the distal side of the anal canal shows a complex component corresponding to the the external sphincter and levator muscles (Kaiser and Reuter 1976). The hypotonicity of the external sphincter and anal canal were seen more frequently in open spina bifida patients who had severe spinal cord lesions, and more frequently with sacral lesions. This suggests that the nerves stemming from the sacral spinal cord play a significant role in the motor activity of the anal canal.

Examination of the anorectal pressure profile and the clinical assessment indicates that clinical status tends to deteriorate in both open and closed forms of spina bifida as the degree of hypotonicity of the muscles of the anal increases. It is therefore possible to make a rough assessment, on the evidence of the anorectal pressure profile, regarding the degree of urgency with which defecational management is required.

It is well known that the RIR in cases of spina bifida is quite similar to that in normal subjects (Ahran 1971; Meunier et al. 1976; Meunier and Mollard 1977; White and Shaker 1974). Characteristics of the reflex in spina bifida are as follows: (a) the amplitude of the basal rhythmical wave is extended and the reflex exaggerated; and (b) the reflex has a lower threshold value. Approximately 70% of closed spina bifida cases showed a normal reflex while more than half of the open spina bifida cases presented a pathological reflex with exaggerated patterns. The occurrence of the reflex even in spinal cord lesions such as spina bifida strongly suggests that it is a local reflex through the intraluminal plexus. However the presence of an exaggerated reflex in spina bifida may be evidence to assume that the spinal component plays a certain role in the RIR.

Meunier et al. (1976) and Meunier and Mollard (1977) have suggested that although the mechanism of the RIR may be due mainly to the function of the intramural plexus, this activity is modulated by the sacral cord. Ihara and Takahira (1984) have demonstrated in experiments on dogs with chronic sacral denervation that a similar enhancement of the reflex, and of the autonomous reflex activities seen in the spina bifida patients, also occurred in these animals. From sacral nerve stimulation and section experiments, they suggested that it is also possible to assume the existence of some permanent inhibitory components acting on the intraluminal plexus through the sacral nerve.

In spina bifida, the extent of injury of the spinal cord differs from patient to patient. This is particularly true in cases of open spina bifida. Yet, although the level of injury of the spinal cord may be identical in open spina bifida, it is legitimate to assume that the extent of lesion at the root level is not identical. It is essential to give consideration to the viability of a neural plaque and to examine the possibility of communication to the central part of the spinal cord.

For this purpose, we measured the spinal evoked potentials during the closure operation for back lesion (Nakagawa et al. 1985). Unfortunately, however, no adequate data are available at present to permit a close analysis of the relationship between the status of the spinal cord and the patient's anal capability. It is our opinion that further research in this field will make a significant contribution to the elucidation of the mechanism of the reflex and defecation.

References

Ahran P (1971) Technique d'exploration fonctionnelle de la motricité digestive en chirurgie pédiatrique. Ann Chir Infant 12:197–206
Forrest D (1976) Management of bladder and bowel in spina bifida. Clin Dev Med 57:122–154
Ihara N, Takahira E (1984) Regulation of anal canal pressure as revealed by myoelectrical activity of internal anal sphincter. Jpn J Smooth Muscle Res 20:123–135
Kaiser G, Reuter I (1976) Betrachtungen zum anorektalen Druckprofil. Z Kinderchir 19:38–49
Lorber J (1971) Results of treatment of myelomeningocele. Dev Med Child Neurol 13:279–303
Meunier P, Mollard H, Beaujen J de (1976) Manometric studies of anorectal disorders in infancy and childhood: an investigation of the physiology of continence and defecation. Br J Surg 63: 402–407
Meunier P, Mollard H (1977) Control of the internal anal sphincter (manometric study with human subjects). Pflugers Arch 370:233–239
Nakagawa T, Imai K, Murakami M, Inoue S, Maie M (1985) Spinal evoked potentials in infants with myelomeningocele. In: Schramm J, Jones SJ (ed) Spinal cord monitoring. Springer, Berlin Heidelberg New York
White JJ, Shaker I (1974) The management of neurological fecal incontinence. Practical management of meningomyelocele. University Park Press, Baltimore, pp 198–217

Anorectal Motility in Children with Complete Rectal Prolapse

H. Suzuki, S. Amano, K. Matsumoto, and Y. Tsukamoto

Summary

Anorectal manometry, defecography, and ultrasonographic study were performed in 36 children with complete rectal prolapse and 45 age- and sex-matched controls. Anorectal manometry disclosed that there was no significant difference in Pr, Pac, or length of HPZ between patients and controls. The rate of BRC of the smooth muscle of the anal canal and RC were significantly lower in patients. Rectoanal reflex was present in all patients and controls. Defecography and ultrasonographic examination confirmed the hypothesis that rectal prolapse starts initially as an intussusception of the rectum, then fully develops. In 29 cases patients were cured by conservative treatment, but seven patients required surgical treatment. Results of modified Sudeck's operation were, in general, satisfactory.

Zusammenfassung

Anorektale Menometrien, Defäkographien und Ultraschalluntersuchungen wurden bei 36 Kindern mit komplettem Rektumprolaps und 45 alters- und geschlechtsentsprechenden Kontrollen durchgeführt. Die anorektale Manometrie ergab keinen signifikanten Unterschied hinsichtlich des Rektaldruckes, des Druckes im Analkanal und der Länge der Region hohen Druckes bei Patienten und zu Kontrollzwecken Untersuchten. Die Rate der basalen Kontraktionen pro Minute der glatten Analkanalmuskulatur und die rektale Compliance waren bei den Patienten signifikant erniedrigt. Ein rektoanaler Reflex war bei Patienten und Kontrollgruppe nachweisbar. Die Defäkographie und die Ultraschalluntersuchung bestätigten die Hypothese, daß der Rektumprolaps mit einer rektalen Invagination beginnt und sich dann voll ausbildet. 29 Patienten wurden konservativ geheilt, die übrigen 7 bedurften der chirurgischen Therapie. Die Ergebnisse der modifizierten Sudeck-Operation waren im allgemeinen gut.

Résumé

On a effectué des manométries anorectales, des défacographies et des examens par échographie pour 36 enfants présentant un rectocèle complet et pour 45 témoins d'âge et de sexe correspondants. La manométrie anorectale ne décela aucune différence significative en ce qui concerne la pression rectale, la pression dans le canal anal et la longueur de la zone de haute pression entre les patients et les contrôles. La fréquence par minute des contractions basales de la musculature lisse du canal anal et la compliance rectale étaient réduites de façon significative chez les patients. On a pu prouver la présence d'un réflexe recto-anal chez les malades et les témoins. La défacographie et l'échographie ont confirmé l'hypothèse selon laquelle le rectocèle commence par une invagination rectale avant de se constituer définitivement. 29 patients ont été guéris par un traite-

---

Second Department of Surgery, Mie University School of Medicine, 2-174 Edobashi, Tsu City 514, Japan

ment conservateur, les 7 autres ayant dû subir une intervention chirurgicale. Les résultats obtenus avec une technique modifiée de l'opération de Sudeck ont été bons dans l'ensemble.

Introduction

The commonly held view that almost all cases of rectal prolapse in children are of a self-limiting mucosal variety is not correct. Complete rectal prolapse is also seen in the pediatric age group, and a certain proportion of children with this disease require surgical treatment (Küpfer and Goligher 1970; Qvist et al. 1986). However, complete rectal prolapse in young children is a rather rare condition, and there have been only a few reports of anorectal motility in children with this disease (Noguchi and Yano 1982; Suzuki et al. 1985). Furthermore, a physiological rationale for the management of rectal prolapse in children has not yet been established. In this communication, we report the results of anorectal manometry, defecography, and an ultrasonographic study of the motility of the anorectum in children with complete rectal prolapse; we also discuss a physiological rationale for the management of this disease in young children.

Materials and Methods

Patients

During the period from January 1978 through August 1986, 36 children with complete rectal prolapse were treated at the Second Department of Surgery, Mie University Hospital, Tsu-City, Japan. These 36 children and 45 age- and sex-matched controls were the subjects of the present study. The patients consisted of 12 boys and 24 girls; the mean ages at the time of diagnosis were 3 years and 2 months (boys) and 3 years and 1 month (girls). The types of prolapse were as follows: grade I (complete eversion of the whole rectal wall through the anal orifice) in one cases; grade II (intussusception of the rectum with protrusion through the anal orifice) in 16; and grade III (concealed prolapse or intussusception of the rectum without protrusion through the anal orifice) in 19. Symptoms reported at the time of diagnosis were as follows: constipation in 31 (86.1%), straining in 20 (55.6%), protrusion of rectal wall through the anal orifice in 17 (47.2%), anal fissure or bleeding in 12, mucous discharge in 6, abdominal pain in 4, fecal incontinence in 2, and mental retardation in 2 patients.

One patient with grade I prolapse was treated surgically, without any prior conservative treatment. Initially, the remaining 35 patients were treated conservatively. Toilet training without any medication was tried in three patients with grade II prolapse, and all three were cured by this treatment. Laxatives were given to 25 patients. The treatment with laxatives cured 20 patients (14 with grade III prolapse and 6 with grade II prolapse). Five patients with grade II prolapse did

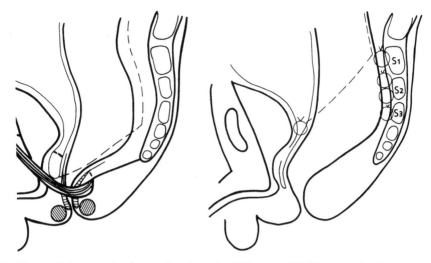

Fig. 1. Schema of the operation for rectal prolapse in children, modified from the description by Sudeck (1922). *Left,* before operation; *right,* after operation

Table 1. Results of modified Sudeck's operation in children with rectal prolapse

Patient number	Age[a]	Sex	Grade of prolapse	Conservative treatment prior surgery[a]	Follow-up period[a]	Outcome
1	6, 10	F	I		0, 6	Satisfactory
2	6, 2	M	II	1, 10	5, 6	Satisfactory
3	2, 3	M	II	0, 4	4, 0	Satisfactory
4	9, 3	F	II	0, 1	2, 10	Satisfactory
5	1, 4	M	II	0, 2	2, 8	Satisfactory
6	4, 8	F	II	0, 2	2, 8	Satisfactory
7	13, 2	M	II	0, 3	1, 7	Satisfactory

[a] Years, months

not respond to the laxatives and were then treated surgically. Laxatives and suppositories were given to seven patients, and these cured six (five patients with grade III prolapse and one with grade II). One patient with grade II prolapse did not respond to laxatives and suppositories and was then treated surgically. The conservative treatment, therefore, cured 10 patients with grade II prolapse and 19 with grade III, but it failed in six patients with grade II prolapse.

Seven patients, in all, were treated surgically, and the results of surgical treatment with the modified Sudeck's operation, shown in Fig. 1, were satisfactory in all cases. The results of the surgical treatment are summarized in Table 1.

Methods of Investigation

Anorectal manometry with infused side-opening catheters was performed in all patients and controls. Rectal pressure (Pr), anal-canal pressure (Pac), length of high-pressure zone (HPZ), rate of basal rhythmic contractions (BRC) of the smooth muscle of the anal canal per minute, rectal compliance (RC), and rectoanal reflex were determined as described previously (Suzuki et al. 1980a, b). Anorectal manometry was performed before and after surgery in six out of seven patients treated surgically.

Defecography was performed in 32 children with complete rectal prolapse. There were 8 boys and 24 girls. The mean ages were 3 years and 2 months (boys) and 3 years and 3 months (girls). The examination was also performed in 30 out of 45 controls. After the instillation of 100–500 ml (100% w/v) barium sulfate, motility of the anorectum was monitored on an X-ray television system (BV X-Ray TV System, Toshiba, Tokyo) in a lateral view and recorded on video tapes (Videocassette KCA-60B, Sony, Tokyo) with a recording system (X-Ray Videocassette Recorder VO-581X, Sony, Tokyo).

An ultrasonographic examination of the motility of the anorectum was performed in seven patients and two controls. The patients were three boys and four girls. The mean ages of patients were 6 years and 10 months (boys) and 3 years and 5 months (girls). Motility of the anorectum at rest and at straining was visualized with a transrectal ultrasonographic probe (UST-675-5, Aloka, Tokyo) attached to an Echo camera (SSD-256, Aloka, Tokyo).

All examinations were performed after informed parental consent had been obtained.

The results are expressed as means ± SD, where applicable. Statistical significance was determined by Student's t test, and values less than $P = 0.05$ were considered to be significant.

Results

Anorectal Manometry

The results of anorectal manometry in 36 children with complete rectal prolapse and in 45 age- and sex-matched controls are given in Table 2. There was no significant difference in the mean values on Pr, Pac, and HPZ between patients and controls. Mean values of BRC and RC were, however, significantly lower in patients than in controls. Rectoanal reflex was present in all patients and controls. There was no difference in the reflex pattern between patients and controls, as shown in Fig. 2. Profiles of resting pressure of the anorectum in each patient are shown in Fig. 3, with their normal values (means ± SD of controls). Pr was within the normal range in 22 patients, higher in 9, and lower in 5. Pac was within the normal range in 33 (91.7%) and lower in 3 patients, one of whom had fecal incontinence. The length of HPZ was within the normal range in 32 patients (88.9%). One in-

Table 2. Results of anorectal manometry

	n	Pr (cm H$_2$O)	Pac (cm H$_2$O)	HPZ (cm)	BRC/ min	RC (ml/cm H$_2$O)
Controls	45	6.5 ± 2.6	81.7 ± 41.2	2.4 ± 0.5	15.8 ± 3.7	7.8 ± 3.3
Patients	36	6.8 ± 3.3	70.6 ± 20.7	2.4 ± 0.4	13.4 ± 2.7	2.6 ± 2.3[a]
Significance		NS	NS	NS	$P<0.01$	$P<0.001$

n, Number of subjects; Pr, rectal pressure; Pac, anal-canal pressure; HPZ, length of high-pressure zone; BRC, rate of basal rhythmic contraction of the smooth muscle of the anal canal; RC, rectal compliance

[a] Rectal compliance was not determined in 2 out of 36 patients with rectal prolapse

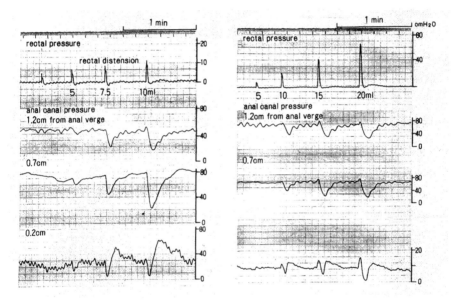

Fig. 2. Rectoanal reflex in patients *(left)* and controls *(right)*. Anal-canal pressure was determined at 0.2, 0.7, and 1.2 cm from anal verge

continent patient had a significantly shortened HPZ. The rate of BRC of the smooth muscle of the anal canal was within the normal range in 22 (61.1%), decreased in 13 (36.1%), and increased in one patient. RC was within the normal range in only two, increased in one, and decreased in 31 out of 34 patients examined (86.1%).

Changes in the profiles of resting pressure of the anorectum before and after surgery were determined in six patients (Fig. 4). Pr increased in four and decreased in two patients after surgery, and four out of six patients showed normal Pac after the operation. Pac increased in four and was unchanged in two patients

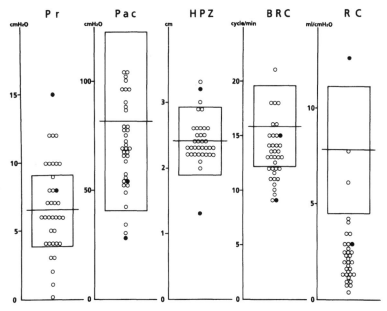

Fig. 3. Profiles of resting pressure of the anorectum in each patient with rectal prolapse. *Boxed columns* indicate means ± SD in the controls. Closed circles, patients with fecal incontinence

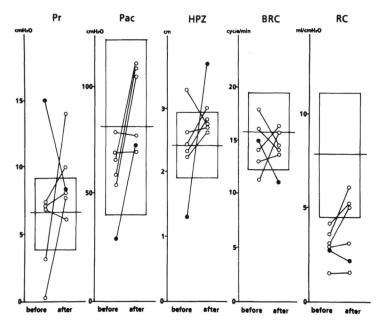

Fig. 4. Profiles of resting pressure of the anorectum before and after surgery. *Boxed columns* indicate means ± SD in the controls

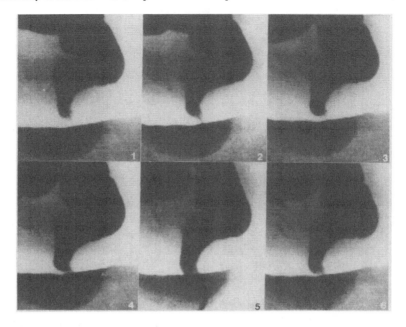

Fig. 5. Defecograms in a normal child

after surgery. All six patients, including one who had fecal incontinence before surgery, showed normal Pac after surgery. The length of HPZ increased in four, was unchanged in one, and decreased in one patient. A remarkable increase in HPZ after surgery was noted in one patient who was incontinent before surgery. The rate of BRC of the smooth muscle of the anal canal increased in two, was unchanged in one, and decreased in three patients after surgery. RC increased to the normal range in three patients after surgery, but it was unchanged in three patients.

Defecography

Defecograms of normal children and of patients are shown in Figs. 5–7. Defecograms of 30 normal children showed that the rectum was filled with the contrast medium, and that the anal canal was closed at rest. Contraction of the rectum, disappearance of the angulation of the rectum, together with opening of the anal canal, occurred during the act of defecation. Defecograms of 32 children with complete rectal prolapse were characterized by the development of an intussusception within the rectum at straining. The intussusception eventually resulted in the complete prolapse of the rectum, with protrusion through the anal orifice in patients with grade II prolapse, while it remained within the rectum in patients with grade III prolapse.

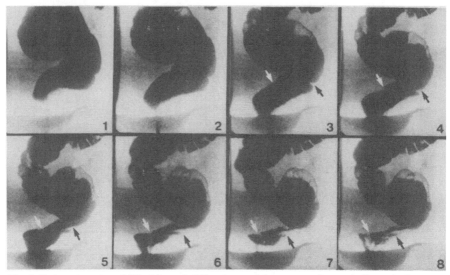

Fig. 6. Defecograms in a child with grade III prolapse of the rectum. *Arrows* indicate the intussusception, which remains within the rectum

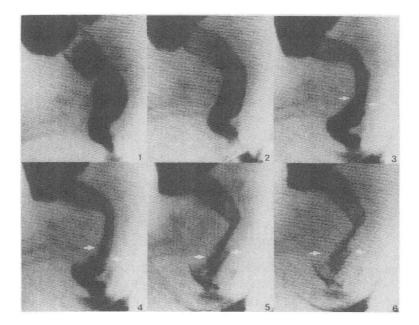

Fig. 7. Defecograms in a child with grade II prolapse of the rectum. The intussusception developed fully and the rectum protruded through the anal orifice

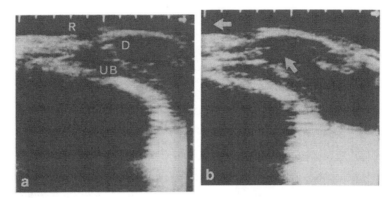

Fig. 8a, b. Ultrasonograms in a child with rectal prolapse at rest (**a**) and at straining (**b**). *R*, Rectal wall; *D*, cul-de-sac; *UB*, urinary bladder. The cul-de-sac deepened on straining and a sliding type of hernia progressed as indicated by the *arrows*

Ultrasonographic Examination

Ultrasonographic examination of the anorectum disclosed that the cul-de-sac was remarkably deeper in patients at rest than in controls, as shown in Fig. 8a. A loose attachment of the rectal wall to the adjacent tissues and the development of a sliding type of hernia in the deep cul-de-sac were characteristic findings in the patients, as shown in Fig. 8b.

Discussion

Results of anorectal manometry disclosed that Pac and the length of HPZ, which represent the resting tone of the anal canal, and the rectoanal reflex, which represents the proper motility of the anal sphincters, did not differ significantly between children with complete rectal prolapse and controls. Noguchi and Yano have also reported that there was no significant difference in the profiles of the resting pressure of the anorectum between seven children with rectal prolapse and seven age-matched controls (Noguchi and Yano 1982). Keighley et al. (1980) carried out anorectal manometry in 45 adult patients with rectal prolapse and found that Pac in patients with rectal prolapse alone did not differ from that in age- and sex-matched controls, but that the pressure in patients with rectal prolapse and fecal incontinence was significantly decreased compared to the controls. Obeid et al. (1979) studied Pac in 20 adult patients with rectal prolapse and found that there was no significant difference in the resting tone of the internal anal sphincter between patients and controls, but that the functional power of the external anal sphincter in patients was significantly decreased. These reports, together with the results of the present study, suggest that the sphincter function of children with rectal prolapse is normal, even in those children with fecal incontinence or abnormal bowel movements, whereas adult patients with abnormal sphincter control or bowel movements have damage in their striated sphincter muscles, probably as a result of long-standing disease (Parks et al. 1977). The cause of significantly decreased RC in children with rectal prolapse is uncertain, but edema and thickening of the rectal wall are often observed in these children and may be the cause of their decreased rectal compliance.

The results of the present defecographic and ultrasonographic studies confirmed the hypothesis that rectal prolapse occurs initially as an intussusception of the rectum, then develops fully (Ripstein and Lanter 1963; Theuerkauf et al. 1970).

The first choice for management of complete rectal prolapse in children is the conservative treatment because the sphincter function in these children is generally normal, and the intussusception of the rectum can be avoided by the elimination of straining by the patients. This concept is supported by the results of our conservative treatment.

However, a certain proportion of patients do not respond to conservative treatment and require surgical treatment. We suggest that the modified Sudeck's operation is effective for the treatment of rectal prolapse in children because the deep cul-de-sac can be closed, the loose attachment of the rectum to the adjacent structure can be reinforced, and the pediatric patients with this disease do not require any procedure to strengthen the anal sphincters. Although the number of patients treated is still small, the results of the modified Sudeck's operation for complete rectal prolapse in children are, in general, satisfactory.

References

Keighley MRB, Makuria T, Alexander-Williams J, Arabi Y (1980) Clinical and manometric evaluation of rectal prolapse and incontinence. Br J Surg 67:54–56

Küpfer CA, Goligher JC (1970) One hundred consecutive cases of complete prolapse of the rectum treated by operation. Br J Surg 57:481–487

Noguchi T, Yano H (1982) Investigation of rectal prolapse in childhood: in view of anorectal manometric study before and after treatment. J Jpn Soc Colo-Proctol 35:463–470 (in Japanese)

Obeid SAF, Zidan H, Hassab MA (1979) Anal sphincteric pressure studies in complete rectal prolapse. Dis Colon Rectum 22:342–345

Parks AG, Swash M, Urich H (1977) Sphincter denervation in anorectal incontinence and rectal prolapse. Gut 18:656–665

Qvist N, Rasmussen L, Klaaborg K-E, Hansen LP, Pedersen SA (1986) Rectal prolapse in infancy: conservative versus operative treatment. J Pediatr Surg 21:887–888

Ripstein CB, Lanter B (1963) Etiology and surgical therapy of massive prolapse of the rectum. Ann Surg 157:259–264

Sudeck P (1922) Rektumprolapsoperation durch Auslösung des Rektum aus der Excavatio sacralis. Zentralbl Chir 20:698–699

Suzuki H, Amano S, Honzumi M, Saijo H, Sakakura K (1980a) Rectoanal pressures and rectal compliance in constipated infants and children. Z Kinderchir 29:330–336

Suzuki H, Matsumoto K, Amano S, Fujioka K, Honzumi M (1980b) Rectoanal pressure and rectal compliance after low anterior resection. Br J Surg 67:655–657

Suzuki H, Amano S, Honzumi M, Iriyama K (1985) Rectoanal pressures and rectal compliance in children with rectal prolapse. Jpn J Surg 15:234–237

Theuerkauf FJ, Bears OH, Hill JR (1970) Rectal prolapse: causation and surgical treatment. Ann Surg 171:819–832

Rectoanal Pressure Studies and Postoperative Continence in Imperforate Anus

N. Iwai, J. Yanagihara, K. Tokiwa, and T. Takahashi

Summary

Functional results after surgical correction of anorectal malformations were assessed on a clinical basis using the Kelly score and by manometric study. In all, 65 patients, aged 5–28 years, were interviewed personally, and 51 of these 65 had manometric studies to evaluate postoperative continence. The manometric study was also performed on 45 normal children as control group. Continent patients characteristically had a marked high-pressure zone, as did the normal subjects. On the other hand, in the patients with fair or poor results, the anorectal pressure profile had no marked high-pressure zone in the anal canal. The presence of normal anal pressure at rest as well as adequate anorectal pressure difference was found to correlate well with continence. In the patients with perineoplasty, the anorectal reflex correlated well with continence, but not in patients treated by abdominoperineal rectoplasty.

Zusammenfassung

Die funktionellen Ergebnisse nach chirurgischer Korrektur anorektaler Fehlbildungen wurden klinisch mit dem Kelly-Score und der Manometrie beurteilt. 65 Patienten im Alter von 5–28 Jahren wurden persönlich befragt und bei 51 dieser 65 Patienten wurden manometrische Untersuchungen zur Bestimmung der postoperativen Kontinenzleistung durchgeführt. Manometrische Untersuchungen wurden ebenfalls bei 45 gesunden Kindern als Kontrollgruppe vorgenommen. Wie gesunde Kinder, hatten kontinente Patienten charakteristischerweise eine ausgeprägte Hochdruckregion. Andererseits wies das anorektale Druckprofil bei Patienten mit mittelmäßigen oder schlechten Ergebnissen keine ausgeprägte Hochdruckregion auf. Es bestand eine enge Korrelation zwischen dem Vorliegen eines normalen analen Ruhedruckes sowie einer adäquaten anorektalen Druckdifferenz und der Kontinenzleistung. Bei Patienten mit Perineoplastik fand sich eine enge Korrelation zwischen anorektalem Reflex und Kontinenzleistung, jedoch nicht bei Patienten, die mit einer abdominoperinealen Rektoplastik behandelt worden waren.

Résumé

Les résultats fonctionnels de la correction chirurgicale des malformations anorectales ont été évalués à l'aide du score de Kelly et de la manométrie. 65 patients, âgés de 5 à 28 ans ont été interrogés individuellement et 51 d'entre eux ont subi des examens manométriques pour déterminer le degré de continence post-opératoire. Un groupe témoin, de 45 enfants sains, a également subi des examens manométriques. Tout comme les enfants en bonne santé, les patients continents présentaient de façon caractéristique une zone de haute pression bien définie. Inversement, les courbes de pression des patients pour lesquels les résultats étaient moyens ou insuffisants, ne présentaient pas de zone de haute pression bien définie. On a constaté un rapport étroit

Division of Surgery, Children's Research Hospital, Kyoto Prefectural University of Medicine, Kamigyo-ku, Kyoto 602, Japan

entre la présence d'une pression anale normale de repos ainsi que d'une différence de pression anorectale adéquate et le degré de continence. Chez les patients avec périnéoplastie, il existe un rapport étroit entre réflexe anorectal et degré de continence, ce qui n'est pas le cas des patients avec rectoplastie abdominopérinéale.

The main object after repair of anorectal malformation is the achievement of fecal continence. Functional results have been assessed mainly on a clinical basis. More recently, objective assessment of continence by manometric study has been added for the complete evaluation of these patients.

This paper describes the clinical and manometric assessment of bowel function after surgical correction of anorectal malformations and the correlation between these two assessments.

Materials and Methods

A total of 139 patients with anorectal malformations were treated from 1960 to 1986 in the First Department of Surgery and Division of Surgery, Children's Research Hospital, Kyoto Prefectural University of Medicine. There were 67 patients (54 males and 13 females) with high-type, 21 patients (13 males and 8 females) with intermediate-type, and 51 patients (34 males and 17 females) with low-type malformations. Of these 139 patients, 65 aged 5–28 years, were interviewed personally, and 51 of these 65 had manometric studies to evaluate postoperative continence. The anorectal manometric study was also performed on 45 normal children, aged 5–11 years (mean, 6 years and 3 months), as a control group.

The usual operative procedure in this department has been a colostomy for the high and intermediate types in the neonatal period, followed by abdominoperineal rectoplasty. The low type of anomaly has been treated by neonatal perineoplasty.

Manometric Study. The probe was filled with water before the examination but was not perfused during the examination. This apparatus was connected to a transducer (Toyo Baldwin Co., Ltd), and the pressure was recorded on a polygraph. Zero pressure, used throughout this study, was determined by recording atmospheric pressure at the anal margin.

The anorectal resting pressure was first recorded (in centimeters) by withdrawing the probe, which was introduced 8 cm above the anal margin. The probe was then set up to locate pressure receptors in the high-pressure zone after examination of the anorectal pressure profile. At this position, the pesence or absence of an anorectal reflex was determined by distending the balloon in the rectum for 10 s.

Clinical Assessment. Clinical assessment of functional results followed the Kelly score system (Kelly 1969); this is based on three criteria: (a) control of feces and bowel habits, (b) fecal staining, and (c) sling action of the puborectal muscle. The results were classified as good (scores 5, 6), fair (3, 4), and poor (0–2).

Results

Clinical Assessments. Of the 23 patients with low-type anomalies, 21 (91%) had good control, and of the 16 patients with intermediate-type anomalies, 10 (63%) achieved good control (Table 1). Of the 26 patients with high-type anomalies, however, only 8 (31%) had good control, and others had fair or poor control.

Anorectal Resting Pressure. A total of 30 patients with good results (11 after staged abdominoperineal rectoplasty for high-type anomalies and 19 after perineoplasty for low-type anomalies) had the same anorectal pressure profile, with a high-pressure zone in the anal canal, as did normal subjects (Table 2). The values for anal resting pressure and anorectal pressure difference were not significantly different from those of normal subjects.

Sixteen patients with fair results (14 of staged abdominoperineal rectoplasty and 2 of perineoplasty) had a less prominent high-pressure zone in the anal canal. The values for anal pressure and anorectal pressure difference were significantly lower ($P < 0.05$) than those in patients with good results and those of normal subjects. However, anal-canal length was identical with that of normal subjects.

In five patients who had undergone staged abdominoperineal rectoplasty, the anorectal pressure profile showed a slight radial change and did not have such a high-pressure zone as was found in the anal canal of normal subjects. Anorectal

Table 1. Functional results and type of anorectal malformations

	Procedure	Number of patients	Functional results		
			Good	Fair	Poor
High type	Staged abdominoperineal rectoplasty	26	8 (31%)	13 (50%)	5 (19%)
Intermediate type	Staged abdominoperineal rectoplasty	11	5 } 10 (63%)	5 } 5 (31%)	1 } 1 (6%)
	Perineoplasty	5	5	0	0
Low type	Perineoplasty	23	21 (91%)	2 (9%)	0

$P < 0.01$

Table 2. Clinical assessment and manometric study of anorectal structures in anorectal malformations after reconstructive surgery (means ± SD)

Functional results	Procedure	Number of patients	Rectal pressure (cm H$_2$O)	Anal pressure (cm H$_2$O)	Anorectal pressure difference (cm H$_2$O)	Anal canal length (cm)
Good	Staged abdominoperineal rectoplasty	11	8.1 ± 1.3	20.1 ± 2.3[a]	15.7 ± 2.2[a]	1.9 ± 0.3
	Perineoplasty	19	7.3 ± 0.7	22.0 ± 1.5[a]	16.4 ± 0.8[a]	1.5 ± 0.4
Fair	Staged abdominoperineal rectoplasty	14	7.2 ± 0.8	13.2 ± 1.6[a]	8.2 ± 0.9[b]	1.5 ± 0.3
	Perineoplasty	2	9.0	18.0	9.5	1.0
Poor	Staged abdominoperineal rectoplasty	5	8.0 ± 1.2	10.1 ± 1.6	4.8 ± 0.7[b]	1.5 ± 0.5
Normal subjects		45	8.9 ± 0.5	23.5 ± 0.8	17.0 ± 0.7	1.6 ± 0.1

[a] $P<0.05$
[b] $P<0.01$

Table 3. Relationship between clinical assessment and the anorectal reflex

Clinical assessment	Procedure	Number of patients	Anorectal reflex Present	Anorectal reflex Absent
Good	Staged abdominoperineal rectoplasty	11	4	7
	Perineoplasty	19	17 } 21 (70%)	2 } 9 (30%)
Fair	Staged abdominoperineal rectoplasty	14	3	11
	Perineoplasty	2	1 } 4 (25%)	1 } 12 (75%)
Poor	Staged abdominoperineal rectoplasty	5	0	5 (100%)

$P<0.01$

pressure difference in the five patients with poor results was 4.8 ± 0.7 cm H_2O; this value was significantly ($P < 0.01$) lower than that in patients with fair results.

Relationship Between Clinical Assessment and the Anorectal Reflex. Of the 30 patients with good results, 21 (70%) had an anorectal reflex, while of the 16 patients with fair results only 4 (25%) did (Table 3). None of the five patients with poor results showed the presence of an anorectal reflex. It is noteworthy that of the 11 patients with good results after staged abdominoperineal rectoplasty, only four had an anorectal reflex, and in the remaining seven patients this reflex could not be observed.

Discussion

The clinical results in patients with imperforate anus in this series are in agreement with most of those in previous reports (Schärli and Kiesewetter 1969; Taylor et al. 1973). The incidence of good results and adequate continence was extremely high in patients with low-type anomalies and low in those with high-type anomalies. These data indicate that patients with low-type anomalies treated with perineoplasty are more likely to be continent, while patients with high-type anomalies treated with abdominoperineal rectoplasty have more problems with continence. It is our belief, as stated also by Nixon and Puri (1977), that the basic reason for the marked difference between the results of high- and low-type anomaly groups is the absence of a functional internal sphincter in the former, with only a rudimentary external sphincter and puborectal muscle left for achieving continence.

Continence after reconstructive surgery for anorectal malformations is related to multiple factors. The present manometric investigations have shown that good clinical results after perineoplasty or abdominoperineal rectoplasty are associated with a normal function of the rectum. This was demonstrated not only by the presence of a normal anorectal pressure profile but also by the presence of an anorectal reflex.

The anorectal pressure profile, observed in all of the patients with adequate continence, characteristically had a marked high-pressure zone, as was the case in the normal subjects. On the other hand, in patients with fair or poor results, the anorectal pressure profile had no marked high-pressure zone in the anal canal, and both the anal resting pressures and the anorectal pressure differences were significantly lower than in those of the continent patients, as well as in those of normal subjects. Thus, the presence of normal anal pressure at rest as well as adequate anorectal pressure difference was found to correlate well with continence subsequent to surgery for anorectal malformations.

The anorectal reflex was observed in 17 of the 19 patients who had adequate continence following perineoplasty while it was demonstrated in only 4 of the 11 patients who had continence after staged abdominoperineal rectoplasty. In addition, it was noted that a reflex was present in four patients who had some degree of incontinence after surgery for a low or an intermediate type of anomaly. These results indicate that in patients with perineoplasty the reflex is correlated well with continence but not in patients treated by abdominoperineal rectoplasty. Accordingly, it seems that the reflex is not essential to achieve continence, at least in patients treated by abdominoperineal rectoplasty.

Arhan et al. (1976) have previously reported that on manometrical grounds, fecal continence is related to multiple factors, such as the presence of an anorectal reflex and adequate length of anal resistance, represented by anal resting pressure. In the present study, it is also true that the presence of a normal anal resting pressure is essential to achieve continence. However, the anorectal reflex in the high type does not necessarily correlate well with continence. Thus, normal anal resting pressure and an adequate anorectal pressure difference in a high-type lesion are more important factors relating to continence after reconstructive surgery for anorectal malformations.

References

Arhan P, Faverdin C, Devroede G, Dubois F, Coupris L, Pellerin D (1976) Manometric assessment of continence after surgery for imperforate anus. J Pediatr Surg 11:157–166

Kelly JH (1969) Cineradiography in anorectal malformations. J Pediatr Surg 4:538–546

Nixon HH, Puri P (1977) The results of treatment of anorectal anomalies: a thirteen to twenty-two year follow-up. J Pediatr Surg 12:27–37

Schärli AF, Kiesewetter WB (1969) Imperforate anus: anorectosigmoid pressure studies as a quantitative evaluation of postoperative continence. J Pediatr Surg 4:694–704

Taylor I, Duthie HL, Zachary RB (1973) Anal continence following surgery for imperforate anus. J Pediatr Surg 8:497–503

Part II
Motility Disturbances of the Gut

Preface

Improved diagnostic procedures, such as rectoanal manometry, electromyography, and histochemical staining of biopsy specimens, have enhanced our knowledge of motility disturbances of the gut. However, in some of these disorders, such as neuronal intestinal dysplasia, small left colon syndrome, chronic intestinal pseudo-obstruction, and other rare clinical entities, we are still only just beginning to understand the underlying mechanisms. This volume of *Progress in Pediatric Surgery* deals with the state of the art in pathophysiological, diagnostic, and, if possible, therapeutic insights into these often only very recently acknowledged disorders.

We greatly appreciate the work of Prof. Jotaro Yokoyama of Keio University, Tokyo, Japan, as guest editor of this volume; he has collected highly valuable papers on constipation and fecal incontinence in children written by Japanese pediatric surgeons and researchers. We are also very grateful to Prof. Morio Kasai of Sendai, Japan, for having written the foreword.

Dr. THOMAS A. ANGERPOINTNER, Munich/FRG

Electrophysiological Principles of Motility Disturbances in the Small and Large Intestines — Review of the Literature and Personal Experience

A. M. Holschneider

Summary

Motility disturbances of the small and large intestines are based on changes in the smooth-muscle potential, whereby the number of amplitudes and configuration of slow waves and of spike potentials as well as pattern, speed of propagation, and duration of the MMC are of crucial importance.

Whereas the electromechanical principles of intestinal motility are sufficiently known, changes in the electromechanical activity in clinically manifest motility disturbances have as yet not been given due regard. Only recently, electromechanical measurements in the upper gastrointestinal tract and colon were performed in several gastrointestinal diseases of internal medicine. In the small intestine, changes in slow waves, spike potentials, and the MMC could be disclosed which are typical for hyperthyrosis, hypothyrosis, irritable bowel syndrome, bacterial diarrhea, primary and secondary intestinal pseudo-obstruction, short-bowel syndrome, postoperative bowel atonia, mechanical bowel obstruction, vagotomy, and diabetic enteropathy with disturbed gastric emptying.

Regarding the colon, a disturbance in the electromechanical characteristics was found in irritable bowel syndrome, bacterial overgrowth in the small bowel, chronic constipation, and idiopathic intestinal pseudo-obstruction, which is probably identical with the clinical picture of adynamic ileus.

Based on a thorough examination of the literature and on own results from electromechanical measurements in children, electromechanical disturbances have been narrowly defined.

Zusammenfassung

Motilitätsstörungen des Dünn- und Dickdarms basieren auf Potentialänderungen der glatten Muskulatur, wobei sowohl die Amplitudenzahl und Konfiguration der „Slow waves" wie der Spikepotentiale sowie, im Dünndarm, die Form, Ausbreitungsgeschwindigkeit und Dauer des „migrating motor complex" (MMC) von entscheidender Bedeutung sind.

Während die elektromechanischen Grundlagen der Dünn- und Dickdarmmotilität hinreichend erforscht sind, wurden Veränderungen der elektromechanischen Aktivität bei klinisch manifesten Motilitätsstörungen bisher kaum beachtet.

Erst in den letzten Jahren hat man im Bereich der inneren Medizin bei einigen gastrointestinalen Erkrankungen elektromechanische Ableitungen des oberen Gastrointestinaltrakts sowie des Kolons und des Rektums durchgefürt.

Dabei konnten für den Bereich des Dünndarms bei den Krankheitsbildern Hyperthyreose, Hypothyreose, irritable Bowelsyndrome, bakterielle Diarrhö, intestinale primäre und sekundäre Pseudoobstruktion, Kurzdarmsyndrom, postoperative Darmatonie, mechanische Darmobstruktion, Vagotomie, diabetische Enteropathie mit Magenentleerungsstörung, typische Veränderungen im Bereich des „slow waves", der Spikepotentiale oder des MMC gefunden werden.

Pediatric Surgical Clinic, City Children's Hospital of Cologne, Amsterdamer Str. 59, D-5000 Köln 60, FRG

Veränderungen der elektromechanischen Charakteristika des Kolons wurden beim „irritable bowel syndrome", der bakteriellen Überwucherung des Dünndarms, der chronischen Obstipation, der intestinalen idiopathischen Pseudoobstruktion, welche wahrscheinlich mit dem Krankheitsbild des adynamen Ileus identisch ist, aufgedeckt.

Aufgrund eines ausführlichen Literaturstudiums und einiger Ergebnisse elektromechanischer Ableitungen bei Kindern werden die elektromechanischen Veränderungen genauer umrissen.

Résumé

Les troubles de la motilité de l'intestin grêle et du côlon sont dus à des variations de potentiel de la musculature lisse. Le nombre d'amplitudes, la configuration des ondes lentes, des potentiels des pointes-ondes particulièrement ainsi que la forme, la vitesse de propagation et la durée du "migrating-motor-complex, MMC" dans l'intestin grêle sont d'une importance capitale.

Alors que de minutieuses études ont porté sur les principes électromécaniques régissant la motilité de l'intestin grêle et du côlon, peu de travail a été consacré à l'étude des variations de l'activité électromécanique dans le cas des manifestations cliniques des troubles de la motilité.

Ce n'est qu'au cours de ces dernières années que l'on a commencé, en médecine interne, à effectuer des mesures électromécaniques des voies gastro-intestinales supérieures, du côlon et du rectum.

On a constaté, en ce qui concerne l'intestin grêle, des modifications caractéristiques des ondes lentes, des potentiels de pointes ou de MMC dans le cas des affections suivantes: hyperthyroïdisme, hypothyroïdisme, colopathies par irritabilité, diarrhées bactériennes, pseudo-occlusions intestinales primaires et secondaires, "short bowel syndrome", atonie intestinale postopératoire, occlusion intestinale mécanique, vagotomie, entéropathie diabétique avec troubles de la vidange de l'estomac.

En ce qui concerne le côlon, on a constaté des modifications des caractéristiques électromécaniques dans les cas de colopathie par irritabilité, pullulation microbienne dans l'intestin grêle, constipation chronique, pseudo-occlusion intestinale idiopathique, cette affection étant probablement identique à la manifestation clinique de l'iléus adynamique.

Les modifications électromécaniques sont ensuite décrites en détail.

Introduction

During recent years, electromanometric and electromyographic measurements in the upper and lower gastrointestinal tract have increasingly been performed in gastroenterological diseases. These have revealed characteristic changes in electrical and electromechanical activities of the small and large bowels which may partially be attributed to distinct clinical entities.

Since electrophysiological investigations of gastrointestinal motility have as yet been scarcely carried out in pediatrics, the author's experiences and a review of the literature will provide a survey of the results to date and of the consequences for differential diagnosis of motility disturbances.

Electrical Activity

Intestinal motility is based on changes of smooth-muscle potentials which occur if a threshold of depolarization is achieved in smooth-muscle cells. In the overall

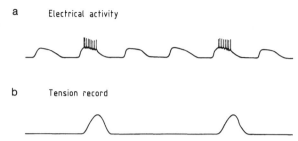

Fig. 1a, b. Slow waves, spikes, and contractions over time. **a** Electrical activity, collection by intracellular microelectrode. Slow waves express themselves as monophasic depolarization, the depolarization being somewhat faster than the repolarization. On the plateau of depolarization of every third slow-wave spike potential bursts appear. **b** Tension record. The contractions are phase linked with spike potential bursts which in turn are controlled by the slow waves. (From Christensen 1971)

human intestine, sinus wave changes in the membrane potential of the muscularis propria mucosae layer can be demonstrated; these are called electrical control activity (ECA), or slow waves, due to their low frequency of 12 cycles/min in the duodenum, 8 cycles/min in the terminal ileum, and 6 cycles/min in the colon. Additional humoral, neuronal, and mechanical stimuli cause a strong depolarization and trigger the so-called spike potentials, or electrical response activity (ERA), on the plateau of slow waves, thus causing a contraction (Bülbring et al. 1970; Gillespie 1968; Christensen 1971; Fig. 1).

The decline in frequency of slow waves from the duodenum to the terminal ileum represents, therefore, the underlying principle of a regular propulsive motility. In the proximal colon the frequency of slow waves declines further to 2–3 cycles/min, increases to 5–6 cycles/min in the descending colon, and stays at 4–8 cycles/min (on average 6) in the rectum. Slow-wave frequency in the rectum has values above average, of 18–24 cycles/min, thus effecting a retrograde peristalsis (Christensen 1971; Holschneider and Metzler 1974; Wienbeck and Altaparmacov 1980).

Electromechanical Rhythm

In the fasting person, slow and fast waves of the smooth-muscle cells, i.e., and ERA, are closely linked to each other, giving rise to an electromechanical rhythm which can be divided into three phases (Fig. 2): This begins with a period of short motoric activity, the so-called activity front, or phase 3, of the migrating motor complex (MMC). Phase 1, a refractory period, follows which is characterized by slow waves without spike potentials and without any motoric activity. Phase 2 then shows irregular slow waves and spike potentials and hence irregular contractions. Phase 2 is followed by phase 3. In this interdigestive, the contractions of phase 3 move from the proximal to the distal small bowel at a speed of 7 cm/min.

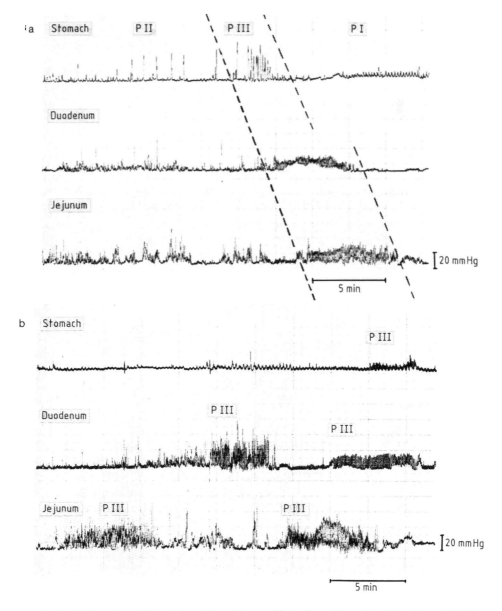

Fig. 2a, b. Normal and disturbed motility of the small intestine. **a** Normal motility. Phase 2 (P II) of the interdigestive MMC is followed by a typically phase-shifted phase 3 (P III), which is of shorter duration but more pronounced in the stomach and of longer duration in the duodenum and jejunum. Thereafter, a regular phase 1 (P I) without motoric activity ensues in all three collection sites. **b** Disturbed motility. Uncoordinated activity with phase 2 nearly completely absent and only hinted in the jejunum between one phase 3 and the next. Phase 3 of the MMC is not regularly phase shifted but rather retrograde (vomiting). In the stomach only a rest period (phase 1) and a hinted phase 3 can be seen. No coordinated time relationship is seen between stomach, duodenum, and jejunum. (By courtesy of Prof. M. Wienbeck, Medizinische Klinik und Poliklinik of the University of Düsseldorf)

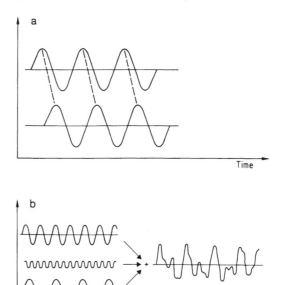

Fig. 3. Diagrammatic representation of electrical activity in the small intestine (**a**) and the large intestine (**b**). **a** Electrical activity is phase controlled (as in Figs. 1, 2a). Electrical waves of constant frequency show a constant phase shift. These slow membrane potential fluctuations of the electrical control activity are the prerequisite for a coordinated bowel movement (myoelectrical control system) and for the impulse-like spike bursts of the smooth-muscle cells. *Spikes,* electrical response activity. **b** Membrane potential fluctuations in the colon show no constant phase shift and are not linked to each other. An irregularly shaped electrical control activity arises from a superimposition of fluctuations of different frequencies. (From Lux et al. 1983)

Period duration of the MMC is about 90 min. When an MMC arrives at the terminal ileum, a new MMC is released from the upper gastrointestinal tract (Vantrappen et al. 1979).

There is a constant phase shift of undulating membrane potentials in the craniocaudal direction in the small intestine, however no phase shift is found in the large intestine, and the several undulating membrane potentials superimpose themselves upon each other, resulting in varying forms of slow waves (Figs. 3, 4). The slow undulation of membrane potentials seems to be coordinated temporarily in the middle of colon so that transitory peristalsis occurs in the transverse and upper descending colon (Lux et al. 1983).

However, discharge patterns are uncoordinated in the proximal and distal colon, causing predominantly segmental contractions in the ascending colon and the rectum. There, short spike discharges signal fast phasic contractions of the ring musculature (Fig. 5), whereas long-lasting spike bursts characterize tonic, slow, short-term, and untransmitted contractions.

These three wave types are thus the slow waves with an average frequency of 6 cycles/min, the short-term spike potentials with a duration of less than 10 s, and the long-term spike potentials with a duration of more than 10 s. In addition to these, however, electrical contraction complexes with a frequency of 25–40 cycles/min, responsible also for tonic continuous contractions, have been described by Sarna et al. (1982; Table 1). We observed such discharge frequencies also in the internal anal sphincter muscle and regarded them as being responsible for the con-

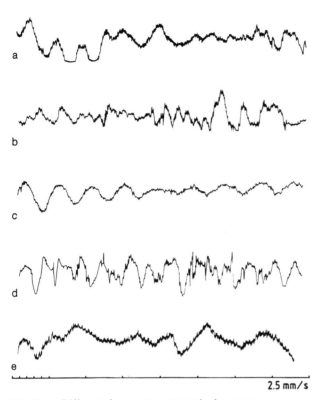

Fig. 4. a–e Different slow waves patterns in the rectum

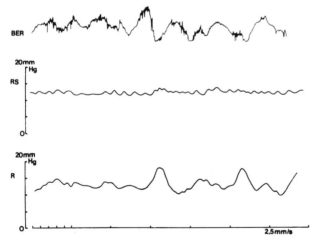

Fig. 5. Extracellular collection of electrical activity from the descending colon. Typical slow waves with spike potentials and phase-coordinated contractions in the rectum. *BER*, basal electrical rhythm; *RS*, rectosigmoid; *R*, rectum

Table 1. Electromechanical characteristics of the colon

Myography	Characteristics	Manometry
Slow waves (electrical control activity)	Frequency 2–9 cycles/min; permanent; different duration and frequency	No mechanical counterpart
Short spike bursts (discrete electrical response activity)	Action potentials of short duration (under 10s); partly periodic with corresponding slow-wave frequency	Short, fast, phasic, partly rhythmic contractions; predominantly in the proximal colon
Long-spike bursts (continuous electrical response activity)	Action potentials of long duration (over 10s); no periodicity; no connection with slow waves	Tonic, slow contractions; no conduction; predominantly in the descending colon
Electrical contraction complex (contractile electrical complex)	Sinusoidal waves; frequency 25–40 cycles/min	Tonic contractions; proximally and distally conducted

(From Sarna et al. 1982)

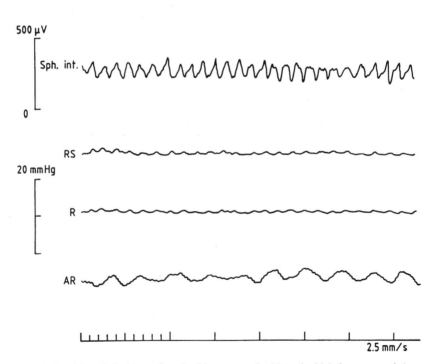

Fig. 6. Electrical activity of the internal anal sphincter muscle. Note the high frequency of slow waves and the missing spike potentials. *SPH. INT.*, Internal sphincter; *RS*, rectosigmoid; *R*, rectum; *AR*, anorectum

tinuous contraction of this organ (Holschneider 1974; Fig. 6). According to Sarna et al. (1980, 1982), however, these electrical wave complexes can also occur in the colon and be conducted proximally and distally, thus potentially causing large mass movements.

Motility Disturbances in the Small and Large Intestines

Although the physiological principles of motility of the small and large bowels have been investigated extensively, consideration has only recently been given to the question of how far motility disturbances are primarily responsible for various diseases or well-known clinical entities (Lederer and Lux 1983).

Disturbances of the ECA, or slow waves, can be distinguished roughly from those of the ERA, or spike potentials, and those of the MMC. Some diseases, however, may be based on several electromechanical disturbances simultaneously.

Disturbances in slow waves

Disturbances in slow waves are observed in hyper- and hypothyrosis as well as in the irritable-bowel syndrome (Table 2). In hyperthyrosis, the frequency of slow waves is increased, as is the motility index, i.e., wave duration times amplitude per time unit of a manometrically measurable contraction. This causes diarrhea (Christensen et al. 1966). In hypothyrosis, the frequency of slow waves and the motility index are decreased, leading to constipation (Christensen et al. 1964).

The irritable bowel syndrome is characterized by reduced or missing MMCs in the small bowel (Thompson et al. 1979) and a decline in slow-wave frequency to 3 cycles/min in the large bowel (Snape et al. 1976). Clinical signs of the irritable bowel syndrome are either diarrhea or spastic constipation due to the reduction in slow-wave frequency. Characteristically, either state may suddenly develop into the another one. (This disease is also not rarely seen in childhood.) This indicates that the observed disturbances in the MMC or the slow waves may occur secondarily and be triggered by primary factors, such as psyche, hormonal influences, allergic components, or metabolic disorders.

Table 2. Disturbances in slow waves

Disease	Disturbance	Author
Hyperthyrosis	Increase in slow wave frequency and motility index	Christensen et al. (1966)
Hypothyrosis	Decrease in slow-wave frequency and motility index	Christensen et al. (1964)
Irritable-bowel syndrome	Small bowel, reduced or missing MMCs; large bowel, reduced frequency of slow waves	Thompson et al. (1979) Snape et al. (1976)

Electrophysiological Principles of Motility Disturbances in the Small and Large Intestines   133

Table 3. Disturbances in spike activity

Clinical signs	Disturbances	Author
Vomiting	Retrograde, conducted spike complexes	Thompson et al. (1982)
Bacterial diarrhea: invasive bacilli (*Shigella dysenteriae, Escherichia coli, clostridium perfringens,* enterotoxin A)	Repetitive spike complexes (i.e., simultaneous ring contractions)	Burns et al. (1980) Justus et al. (1981) Mathias et al. (1980)
Bacterial diarrhea: noninvasive bacilli (*Vibrio cholerae clostridium difficile, Escherichia coli*)	Fast, aborally migrating spike complexes (i.e., peristaltic contractions)	Justus et al. (1981) Mathias et al. (1980)

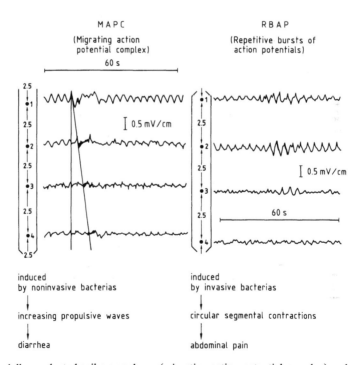

Fig. 7. Fast orthogradally conducted spike complexes (migrating action potential complex) and repetitive spike complexes (repetitive bursts of action potentials) in bacterial diarrhea due to noninvasive bacilli (*left;* accelerated transport of bowel contents) and invasive bacilli (*right;* ring contractions causing abdominal pain). (From Mathias et al. 1976)

Disturbances in Spike Activity

Disturbances in spike activity occur in vomiting and bacterial diarrhea (Table 3). Retrograde migration of spike burst complexes may represent a distinct clinical entity in infants. Such infants present clinically with bile-stained vomiting without any obstructive correlative. These patients occasionally undergo unnecessary laparotomy for roentgenographically or sonographically suspected bowel obstruction, although nothing pathological can be found. Therapy of choice is total parenteral nutrition for several weeks followed by careful, stepwise enteral nutrition via Alfaré. Further investigation must elucidate how far the pathological retrograde migration of spike activity is a sign of maturation disturbance in electromechanical conduction. Also in bacterial diarrhea, repetitive spike complexes associated with multiple simultaneous ring contractions may occur in the terminal ileum due to invasive bacilli such as *Shigella dysenteriae, Escherichia coli, Clostridium perfringens,* or enterotoxin A. Alternatively, fast, aborally migrating spike complexes with peristaltic contractions may occur due to noninvasive bacilli such as *Vibrio cholerae, C. perfringens,* or *E. coli* (Mathias et al. 1980; Justus et al. 1981, 1982; Fig. 7) Gastroenteritis caused by *Versinia bacilli,* which must be included in the differential diagnosis of acute appendicitis for its intense, often spastic abdominal pains, also possibly induces similar repetitive spike complexes in the terminal ileum.

Disturbances in the Interdigestive Migrating Motor Complex

Disturbances in the MMC may be observed under conditions of psychic stress (McCrahe et al. 1982), following vagotomy (Foster et al. 1982), with nicotine uptake (Demol et al. 1983), and in diabetic enteropathy with disturbed gastric emptying (Malagaleda et al. 1980; McNally et al. 1969, Table 4). Moreover, they were described by Remington et al. (1983) in the short bowel syndrome, by Altaparmakov et al. (1985) in postoperative bowel atonia, by Summers et al. (1982) in

Table 4. Disturbances of the interdigestive migrating motor complex (MMC)

Disease	Disturbance	Author
Psychic stress	Suppression of MMC	McCrahe et al. (1982)
Vagotomy	Q complexes with disturbed MMC intervals	Foster et al. (1982) Thompson et al. (1982)
Nicotine uptake	Accelerated conduction of phase 3 of MMC	Demol et al. (1983)
Diabetic enteropathy with disturbed gastric emptying	Pathological Q complexes; anomalous MMC; loss of tone with increase of pathological MMC cycles	Foster et al. (1982) Malagaleda et al. (1980) McNally et al. (1969)

Table 5. Disturbances of the interdigestive migrating motor complex (MMC)

Disease	Disturbance	Author
Short bowel syndrome	Increased frequency of phase 3 of MMC; shortened phase 2	Remington et al. (1983)
Postoperative bowel atonia	Missing MMC	Altaparmakov et al. (1985)
Mechanical bowel obstruction	Partly missing MMC, reduced motility index; Q complexes of high frequency	Summers et al. (1982)
Chagas' disease	Slowed migration speed and duration of phase 3 of MMC	Oliveira et al. (1983)

mechanical bowel obstruction, and by Oliveira et al. (1983) in Chagas' disease (Table 5). MMCs are missing in postoperative bowel atonia, whereas they are slowed down, reduced, or changed in mechanical bowel obstruction and Chagas' disease.

In this context, the short bowel syndrome may be particularly emphasized. Whereas in the colon, normal slow wave cycles only with minimal single spike potentials superimposed upon the plateau of slow waves can be demonstrated in the fasting patient, spike potentials show an increase about 15–20 min following food intake. These spike potentials are significantly increased already after food intake of 1000 calories (Snape et al. 1978, 1979). Interestingly, however, food composition decisively influences spike activity and thus colonic motility. Wright et al. (1980) have shown that fat combined with carbohydrates or protein causes a motility peak after 10–60 min which may be suppressed by a preceding intake of amino acids (Fig. 8). This could mean a therapeutic possibility in the treatment of short bowel syndrome.

Disturbances in the MMC are also observed in intestinal idiopathic pseudo-obstruction, which is possibly identical with the so-called adynamic bowel syndrome, or chronic primary intestinal pseudo-obstruction. This clinical picture has been investigated by numerous groups, but most authors have not found typical interdigestive MMCs (Wienbeck and Erckenbrecht 1983; Summers et al. 1982; Waterfall et al. 1981; Foster et al. 1982). Sarna et al. (1978) attributed this to a hyperpolarization of smooth-muscle cells in the sense of a myogenic idiopathic pseudo-obstruction, whereas Kumpuries et al. (1979) saw neuronal influences with subsequent hypermotility and increased MMC amplitude as responsible for pseudo-obstruction (Table 6).

Secondary pseudo-Obstructions are found following Crohn's disease or sclerodermia (Rees et al. 1982) as well as bacterial overgrowth of the bowel (Vantrappen et al. 1977, 1979). Disturbances in esophageal motility in sclerodermia have long been known; on account of this, measurement of esophageal pressure may be a diagnostic tool if visceral affection is suspected.

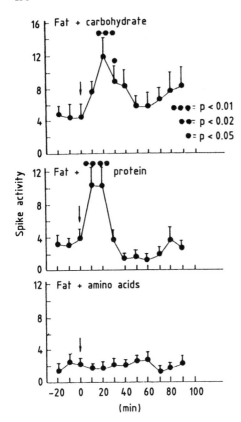

Fig. 8. Colonic motility following fat carbohydrate, protein, and amino acid uptake. (From Wright et al. 1980)

Table 6. Disturbances in the interdigestive migrating motor complex (MMC)

Clinical signs	Disturbance	Author
Intestinal idiopathic pseudo-obstruction	No typical MMC; increased Q complexes	Summers et al. (1982) Kumpuries et al. (1979) Waterfall et al. (1981)
	Missing phases 1 and 2	Foster et al. (1982)
	Jejunal retroperistalsis	Waterfall et al. (1981)
	Hyperpolarization of smooth-muscle cells (myogenic form)	Sarna et al. (1978)
	Hypermotility, MMC with superelevated amplitude (neuronal form)	Kumpuries et al. (1979)
Secondary pseudo-obstruction in sclerodermia and bacterial overgrowth of the bowel	No MMC (missing phase 3)	Rees et al. (1982) Vantrappen et al. (1977)

Electrophysiological Principles of Motility Disturbances in the Small and Large Intestines   137

Hirschsprung's Disease

Motility disturbances of the small intestine in Hirschsprung's disease have as yet not been investigated. However, our measurements of ECA and ERA in nine children with Hirschsprung's disease have shown that disturbances in the cycle of slow waves are more important pathologically than are changes of spike potentials. Lack of spike potentials on the plateau of slow waves in patients with Hirschsprung's disease, formerly observed by us (Holschneider 1982, 1983), seems to be method dependent, especially as Wood (1973) demonstrated by intracellular measurements in mice with Hirschsprung's disease that spike frequency increases in the aganglionic segment with regard to healthy bowel, exhibiting, however, irregular patterns. This means that the contractions in the aganglionic segment are irregular, too.

Our investigations in nine children with Hirschsprung's disease also revealed irregular slow-wave cycles. Four children had slow waves with more than 12 cycles/min, but only four children had normal frequencies of 5–6 cycles/min, and one patient showed a reduced frequency of 2–3 cycles/min. Moreover, propulsive activities could be observed. The increased slow-wave frequency was similar to that of the internal anal sphincter muscle, expressing an increased contraction readiness of the aganglionic segment (Fig. 9). One child with so-called adynamic bowel syndrome exhibited slow-wave cycles with a normal frequency of 9 cycles/min in the small intestine and of 6 cycles/min in the large intestine. However, this

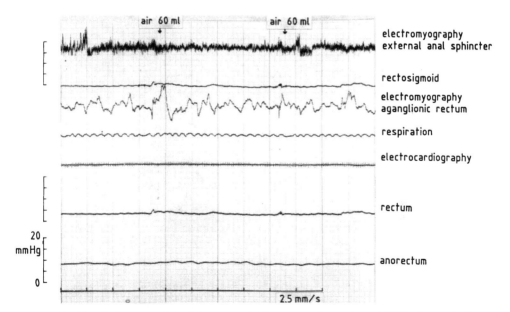

Fig. 9. Electrical presentation of slow waves in the rectum of a patient with Hirschsprung's disease. Irregular slow waves without spike potentials. EMG of the external anal sphincter muscle

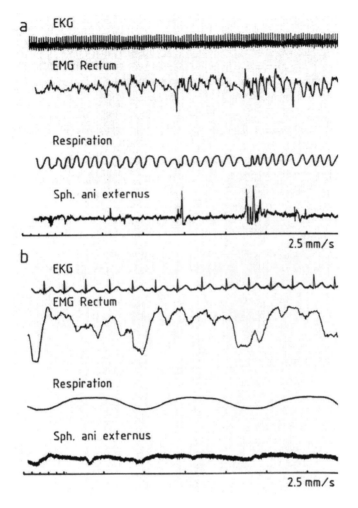

Fig. 10a, b. Electrical activity of the rectum in a newborn with enterocolitis. **a** Adynamic bowel syndrome. High frequency of irregular slow waves, partly solitary, but associated with the slow-wave plateau spike potentials. **b** Low-frequency slow waves condensed as three or four cycles in ultraslow electrical fluctuations (respiration dependent?)

child had an absence of any spike complexes in the overall gut. Another patient showed pathological slow-wave complexes of 3–5 cycles/min in the transverse colon which seemed to be condensed in units (Fig. 10). And another child with neuronal colonic dysplasia exhibited high-frequency slow waves in the region of the right colonic flexure, as a sign of an obstructive motility disturbance.

Conclusions

The review of the literature and our own measurements reported here make evident that primary changes in gastrointestinal motility account for certain clinical pictures of bowel obstruction and diarrhea. On the other hand, there are a large number of electrophysiological disturbances which influence bowel motility secondary to primary diseases. Therefore, further electrophysiological investigations are necessary for a more profound clarification of many so far unknown pathophysiological interrelationships in motility disturbances without a pathological-anatomic substrate. It may be possible that electromechanical causes of the adynamic bowel syndrome, the megacystis-microcolon-intestinal-hyperperstalsis syndrome, the meconium blockage syndrome, the small left colon syndrome, and some other motility disturbances can be clarified only this way.

References

Altaparmakov I, Erckenbrecht JF, Wienbeck M (1985) Modulation of the adrenergic system in the treatment of postoperative bowel atonia. Scand J Gastroenterol 20:135–142

Bülbring E, Brading A, Jons A, et al (1970) Smooth muscle. Edward, London

Burns TW, Mathias JR, Martin JL, Carlson GM, Shields RP (1980) Alteration of myoelectric activity of small intestine by invasive *Escherichia coli*. Am J Physiol 238:57–62

Christensen J (1971) The controls of gastrointestinal movements: some old and new views. N Engl J Med 285:85–98

Christensen J, Schedel HP, Clifton J (1964) The basic electrical rhythm of human duodenum in normal subjects and in patients with thyroid disease. J Clin Invest 43:1659–1665

Christensen J, Schedel HP, Clifton J (1966) The small intestinal basic electrical rhythm (slow wave) frequency gradient in normal man and in patients with a variety of disease. Gastroenterology 50:309–315

Demol P, Hotz J, Singer MV, Dipp M, Goebel H (1983) Erhöhte Ausbreitungsgeschwindigkeit des interdigestiven Motorkomplexes (IMC) bei Rauchern. Z Gastroenterol 11:429–430

Foster GE, Arden-Jones JR, Evans DF, Beatti A, Hardcastle JD (1982) Abnormal jejunal motility in gastrointestinal disease: The Q-complex. In: Winbeck M (ed) Motility of the digestive tract. Raven, New York, pp 427–432

Gillespie JS (1968) Electrical activity in the colon. In: Handbook of physiology, sect 6, alimentary canal IV. American Physiological Society, Bethesda

Holschneider AM (1974) Elektromyographische Untersuchungen der Musculi sphincter ani externus und internus in bezug auf die anorektale Manometrie. Langenbeck's Arch Chir 333:303–312

Holschneider AM (1982) Hirschsprung's disease. Hippokrates, Stuttgart, pp 72–86

Holschneider AM (1983) Elektromanometrie des Enddarmes: Diagnostik und Therapie der Inkontinenz und chronischen Obstipation, 2nd edn. Urban and Schwarzenberg, München, pp 6–24

Holschneider AM, Metzler EM (1974) Manometrische Studien zur anorektalen Kontinenz im Kindesalter. Brun's Beitr Klin Chir 221:14–20

Justus PG, Mathias JR, Martin JL, et al (1981) Myoelectric activity in the small intestine in response to *Clostridium perfringens* and enterotoxin: correlation with histologic findings in an in vivo rabbit model. Gastroenterology 80:902–906

Justus PG, Martin JL, Goldberg DA, et al (1982) Myoelectric effects of *Clostridium deficile*: motility – altering factors distanced from its cytotoxin and enterotoxin in rabbits. Gastroenterology 83:836–843

Kumpuries DD, Brannan PG, Goyal RK (1979) Characterisation of motor activity in the jejunum of normal subjects and two patients with idiopathic intestinal pseudoobstruction syndrome (abstr). Gastroenterology 76:177

Lederer PC, Lux G (1983) Dünndarmmanometrie. In: Winbeck M, Lux G (eds) Gastrointestinale Motilität, klinische Untersuchungsmethoden. Edition Medizin, Weinheim, pp 65–74

Lux G, Lederer PC, Ellermann A (1983) Manometrie und Elektromyographie im Rektosigmoidbereich. In: Winbeck M, Lux G (eds) Gastrointestinale Motilität, klinische Untersuchungsmethoden. Edition Medizin, Weinheim, pp 91–104

Malagaleda JR, Rees WDW, Mazzotta LJ, Go VLW (1980) Gastric motor abnormalities in diabetic and postvacotomy gastroparesis: effect of metoclopramide and bethanechol. Gastroenterology 78:286–293

Mathias JR, Carlson GM, DiMarino AJ, Bertiger G, Morton HE, Cohen S (1976) Intestinal myoelectric activity in response to live *Vibrio cholerae* and cholera enterotoxin. J Clin Invest 58:91–96

Mathias JR, Carlson GM, Martin JL, Shields RP, Formal S (1980) *Shigella dysenteriae* 1 enterotoxin: proposed role in pathogenesis of shigellosis. Am J Physiol 239:382–386

McCrahe S, Younger K, Thompson DG, Wingeate DL (1982) Sustained mental stress alters human jejunal motor activity. Gut 23:404–409

McNally EF, Reinhardt AE, Schwarz PE (1969) Small bowel motility in diabetics. Am J Dig Dis 14:163–169

Oliveira RB, Meninghelli UG, De Godoy RA, et al (1983) Abnormalities of interdigestive motility of the small intestine in patients with Chagas' disease. Dig Dis Sci 28:294–299

Rees WDW, Leigh RJ, Christofides ND, Bloom SR, Turnberg LA (1982) Interdigestive motor activity in patients with systemic sclerosis. Gastroenterology 83:575–580

Remington M, Malagaleda JR, Zinsmeister A, Fleming CR (1983) Abnormalities in gastrointestinal motor activity in patients with short bowels: effect of a synthetic opiate. Gastroenterology 85:629–636

Sarna SK, Daniell EE, Waterfall WE, Lewis TD, Marzio L (1978) Postoperative gastrointestinal electrical and mechanical activities in a patient with idiopathic intestinal pseudoobstruction. Gastroenterology 74:112–120

Sarna SK, Bardakjian BC, Waterfall WE, Lind JF (1980) Human colonic electrical control activity (ECA). Gastroenterology 78:1526–1532

Sarna SK, Latimer P, Campell B, Waterfall WE (1982) Electrical and contractile activity of the human rectosigmoid. Gut 23:698–710

Snape WJ, Carlson GM, Cohen S (1976) Colonic myoelectric activity in the irritable bowel syndrome. Gastroenterology 70:326–330

Snape WJ, Matarazzo SA, Cohen S (1978) Effect of eating and gastrointestinal hormones on human colonic myoelectrical and motor activity. Gastroenterology 75:373–378

Snape WJ, Wright SH, Battle WM, Cohen S (1979) The gastrocolic response: evidence for a neural mechanism. Gastroenterology 77:1235–1240

Summers RW, Anuras S, Green J (1982) Jejunal motility patterns in normal subjects and symptomatic patients with parial mechanical obstruction or pseudoobstruction. In: Wienbeck M (ed) Motility of the digestive tract. Raven, New York, pp 467–470

Thompson DG, Wingate DL, Laidlow JM (1979) Abnormal small bowel motility demonstrated by radio telemetry in a patient with irritable colon. Lancet II:1321–1323

Thompson DG, Ritchie HD, Wingate DL (1982) Patterns of small intestinal motility in duodenal ulcer patients before and after vagotomy. Gut 23:517–523

Vantrappen G, Janssens J, Hellemanns J, Ghoos Y (1977) The interdigestive motor complex of normal subjects and patients with bacterial overgrowth of the small intestine. J Clin Invest 59:1158–1166

Vantrappen G, Janssens J, Peters D, Hellemanns J (1979) The interdigestive complex in health and disease. In: Demling L, Strunz U, Domschke W (eds) Gastrointestinale Motilitätsstörungen, pathophysiologische und klinische Aspekte. (Die gastroenterologische Reihe, Sonderband 1979.) Kali-Chemie Pharma GmbH, Hannover, pp 147–153

Waterfall WE, Cameron GS, Sarna SK, Lewis DT, Daniell EE (1981) Disorganized electrical activity in a child with idiopathic intestinal pseudo-obstruction. Gut 22:77–83

Wienbeck M, Altaparmacov I (1980) Is the internal anal sphincter controlled by a myoelectrical mechanism? Gastrointestinal motility. Raven, New York

Wienbeck M, Erckenbrecht J (1983) Funktionelle Störungen des Dünndarmes. In: Caspary WF (ed) Dünndarm. Springer, Berlin Heidelberg New York, pp 631–639 (Handbuch der inneren Medizin, vol 3, pt 3B)

Wood JD (1973) Electrical activity of the intestine of mice with hereditary megacolon and absence of enteric ganglion cells. Am J Dig Dis 18:477–489

Wright SH, Snape WJ, Battle W, Cohen S, London KL (1980) Effect of dietary components on gastrocolonic response. Am J Physiol 238:232–239

The Practical Significance of Manometry in Pathology of the Rectum and Anorectum

A. F. Schärli

Summary

In practical usage, manometry of the rectum and anorectum has proven reliable in providing reproducible measurements; among these are the relaxation reflex, the anorectal pressure profile, and the squeeze pressure produced by active voluntary contraction of the anorectum. In differential diagnosis, there are three major areas of indication: (a) as a screening method in patients with fecal retention to differentiate between constipation and neural disorder; (b) evaluation of continence after surgery for anal agenesis or sphincter replacement, and (c) work-up of residual symptoms after surgery for Hirschsprung's disease. To date, many manometrically obtainable findings have attained chiefly scientific significance.

Zusammenfassung

In der Praxis hat sich die Manometrie des Rektums und Anorektums als verläßliche Methode erwiesen, bei der Messung
- des Relaxationsreflexes,
- des anorektalen Druckprofiles und
- des Pressdruckes durch aktive Willkürkontraktion des Anorektums

reproduzierbare Ergebnisse zu liefern.
Differentialdiagnostisch lassen sich 3 Hauptindikationen unterscheiden:
- Screeningmethode bei Patienten mit Stuhlretention zur Differenzierung zwischen Obstipation und neuralen Ursachen;
- Beurteilung der Kontinenz nach Operationen bei anorektalen Fehlbildungen oder Sphinkterersatz;
- Abklärung von Residualsymptomen nach Operationen bei M. Hirschsprung.

Viele der Befunde, die mit der Manometrie erhoben wurden, sind heute von großer wissenschaftlicher Bedeutung.

Résumé

En pratique, la manométrie du rectum et de l'anorectum s'est révélé être une méthode fiable, en ce qui concerne:
- la mesure du réflexe de relâchement,
- la mesure du profil de la pression anorectale et
- la mesure de la pression par contraction volontaire et active de l'anorectum,

et donne des résultats reproductibles.
En ce qui concerne le diagnostic différentiel, on distingue trois indications principales:
- dépistage des patients présentant une rétention des selles pour établir une différence entre constipation et troubles neuraux;

Dept. of Pediatric Surgery, Children's Hospital, CH-6000 Luzern 16, Switzerland

- évaluation de la continence après traitement chirurgical de malformations anorectales ou de sphinctéroplastie;
- mise en évidence de symptômes résiduels après opération dans les cas de maladie de Hirschsprung.

Un grand nombre des constatations et résultats obtenus grâce à la manométrie sont aujourd'hui d'une importance scientifique considérable.

The Development of Manometry

In the quest to objectify the results of clinical studies, the use of rectal and anorectal manometry has increased worldwide over the past 20 years. Nonetheless, its routine use is still restricted to relatively few institutions and few indications.

As early as 1877, Gowers (1877) described reflex relaxation of the internal anal sphincter after rectal dilatation. More exact observations of the motor activity of colon and rectum were made by Bayliss and Starling (1899), Cannon (1939), and Templeton and Lawson (1932). Denny-Browne and Robertson (1934) studied the neural control of defecation. Schuster et al. (1965) were the first to describe changes in the internal sphincter reflex in Hirschsprung's disease.

Our own studies (Schärli 1971; Schärli and Kiesewetter 1969) revealed a number of additional processes in the rectum and anorectum:

- Adaptation reaction: Propulsion with mass movement in the rectum is followed by a typical pattern of motion consisting of continually decreasing bowel wall contractions. In this way, the rectum achieves a reservoir function (Fig. 1).

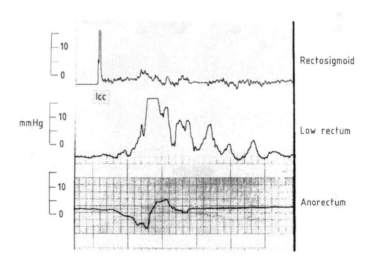

Fig. 1. Rectal adaptation reaction triggered by transport of bowel contents. Rapid pressure increase is followed by gradual pressure decrease. Anorectal pressure rises on arrival of propulsive wave (continence reaction)

- Continence reaction: Simultaneously with the mass movement, a voluntary or involuntary reflex contraction of striated muscle is initiated in the anorectum, preventing stool discharge in both waking and sleeping states (Fig. 2).
- Internal sphincter performance: The circular smooth muscle of the anorectum maintains a substantial pressure barrier in the form of undulating contractions. Stimulation of the rectum by a bolus of water, air, or intrinsic propulsion leads to myogenic reflex relaxation. In this manner, reduction of the pressure barrier becomes a preliminary step in defecation (Fig. 3).

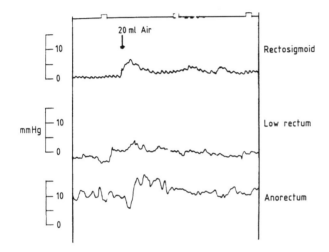

Fig. 2. Continence reaction. Reflex contraction of sphincter complex on arrival of propulsive wave induced by 20 ml air

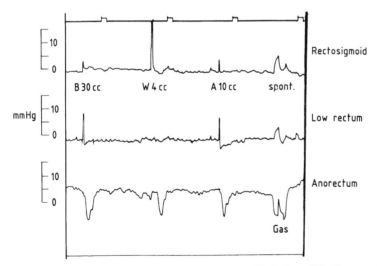

Fig. 3. Relaxation of internal sphincter triggered by balloon (30 ml), water instillation (4 ml), free air (10 ml), or propulsive wave

Table 1. Maturation of the rectum

Stage	Defecation	Stools	Continence reaction	Adaptation reaction	Defecatory reflex	Significance
1	With each propulsive wave	Fluid, not formed, frequent	0	0	0	Incontinence
2	With propulsive waves	Mushy, frequent	Beginning to show	Beginning to show	0	
3	4–8 times per day, under some control	Formed at times	Limited to small waves <10 mmHg	For small mass increase	To low rectum	Partial continence
4	Less frequent, 3–6 times per day	Soft, more or less formed	Complete, except for big waves	Complete	To high rectum	Continence
5	1–2 times per day	Formed, normal consistency	Complete	Complete	To sigmoid colon	

- Induction of defecation: A sensation of fecal urgency at the level of the anorectal ring triggers a propulsive mass movement from the rectosigmoid or rectum. This reflex process is dependent upon intact anorectal sensory innervation and a presently unknown reflex pathway.
- Calculation of continence achievement: Continence achievement can be expressed quantitatively by calculating the propulsive motion and pressure increase in the anorectum (Schärli and Kiesewetter 1969).
- Rectal maturation: After rectal resection, the pulled-through colon assumes the function of a neorectum. Five maturational stages may be observed by registration of the continence reaction, the adaptation reaction, and the course of defecation (Table 1).

Varma and Stephens (1972) have defined anorectal reflex behavior in numerous pathological conditions. Differing findings were observed in meningomyelocele, Hirschsprung's disease, and rectal agenesis, among others. In the same year, Kelly (1972) introduced a scoring system based on clinical and manometric studies to determine the degree of continence. And in 1976, Holschneider and Metzler (1976) characterized the concept of rectal compliance and demonstrated alterations associated with acquired megarectum and congenital megacolon.

Limitations of Manometry

Manometry is carried out using a balloon or probe system to measure a summation effect of pressure changes at one or more sites in the rectum or anorectum. Conclusions as to physiological or pathological conditions in the bowel wall or

Table 2. Alterations in colon activity by various influencing factors

	Colon activity	
	Elevated	Decreased
Physiological	Eating	Sleep
Psychological	Stress	Excitement
Humoral	Gastrin Prostaglandin E_1	Serotonin
Drugs	Neostigmine Morphine (tone)	Atropine
Local	Enema	High-bulk diet
Pathological	Constipation Irritable bowel syndrome Megacolon (ganglionic)	Diarrhea Rectal inertia Megacolon (aganglionic)

sphincter apparatus may be drawn. In practice, however, performance of the technique and interpretation of the results involve certain difficulties:

- Sedation is often necessary in newborns, infants, and young children. Numerous artifacts due to movement or crying affect the validity of the measurements.
- The method is time consuming and requires a patient examiner.
- Up to the present, the measurements have not been internationally standardized.
- Differences in technique (balloon and probe recordings) lead to variable pressure values (Arhan and Faverdin 1971; Schärli 1971).
- Interpretation very often depends on the experience and routine of the examiner.
- Each pressure measurements expresses a summation of complex functions of bowel wall or sphincters, thus limiting conclusions as to individual functions.

In studying colonic activity, it becomes apparent that even changes in physiological conditions may produce elevated or reduced activity: eating, stress, gastrin, neostigmine, or morphine lead to increased activity, while sleep, excitement, serotonin, and atropine decrease it. Under pathological circumstances, bowel activity is increased by constipation or irritable bowel syndrome and decreased by diarrhea or in the aganglionic segment of a megacolon (Table 2; Holschneider 1974; Holschneider et al. 1976; Schärli and Kiesewetter 1969).

Prerequisites for Practical Significance of Manometry

The examination has proved to be of practical significance where reproducible pressure sequences are present, particularly in the anorectal sphincter complex.

Table 3. Quantitating measurements in continence, partial continence, and incontinence

Measurement	Continence	Partial continence	Incontinence
Pressure profile	25 mm Hg	15–25 mm Hg	15 mm Hg
Anorectal length	3–5 cm	2–3 cm	2 cm
Relaxation reflex	Regular (15–30 mm Hg)	Weak, often atypical	Often absent
Active external sphincter contraction	Twofold resting pressure	Ca. 10–20 mm Hg	10 mm Hg
Duration of external sphincter contraction	30–50 s	10–30 s	Under 10 s
Continence reaction	Compensates each propulsion	Does not compensate high propulsive waves	Does not compensate even slight propulsions
Adaptation reaction	Normal	Incomplete	Absent

- The anorectal pressure profile is decreased and shortened in incontinence (Schärli 1983).
- The anorectal relaxation reflex confirms a functioning internal sphincter and is regularly absent in aganglionosis or the neuronal dysplasias (distinction from chronic constipation; Holschneider et al. 1976; Schärli 1972; Schuster et al. 1965).
- Squeeze pressure is absent in pelvic floor paralysis and reduced with muscular incontinence.
- Changes in sphincter activity after corrective surgery or pelvic floor training can be objectified by means of these parameters.

Anorectal Pressure Profile. On pull-through manometry, anorectal resting pressure differs from rectal pressures by around 4–5 cm. Depending on the technique employed, maximal resting pressure is normally over 25 mm Hg, and sphincter length is more than 3.5 cm. Values below 15 mm Hg and less than 2 cm are synonymous with a diagnosis of incontinence (Table 3).

Anorectal Pressure Profile and Squeeze Pressure. Under normal conditions, the pressure profile is approximately doubled by active sphincter contraction. In muscular incontinence, even maximal contractile force is deficient (Fig. 4).

Internal Sphincter Relaxation. While a rudimentary reaction is found with myogenic achalasia, internal sphincter relaxation is generally absent in aganglionic megacolon (Fig. 5; Holschneider 1974).

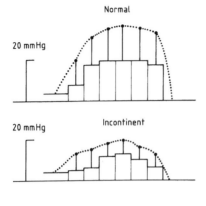

Fig. 4. Anorectal pressure profile and squeeze pressure *(dotted lines)* with normal continence (anorectal profile, 4–5 cm; magnitude, 20 mm Hg; squeeze, twofold) and incontinence (anorectal profile, diminished; magnitude, 20 mm Hg; squeeze, low)

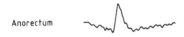

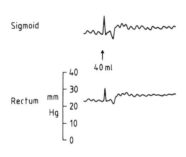

Fig. 5. In Hirschsprung's disease, internal sphincter fails to relax or actually contracts following rectal distention

Significance of Manometry in Characterizing Disorders of the Rectum and Anorectum

Hirschsprung's Congenital Megacolon. In the ganglionic portion of the megacolon, the bowel musculature is hyperperistaltic, and propulsive activity is intact. Propulsion ceases in the transition zone; muscular contractions are almost totally absent, but there is no zone of excessive pressure. The aganglionic segment lacks any propulsive activity, and the internal sphincter reflex to rectal distension is regularly absent. Mass contractions are occasionally elicited spontaneously or by stimulation of the rectal wall, indicating an inability of the bowel musculature for coordination. At times, pressure increases or salvos of spastic contractions are produced (Fig. 6; Schärli 1972, 1982).

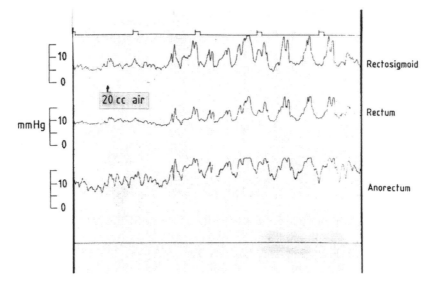

Fig. 6. Mass contractions in aganglionic segment and anorectum in Hirschsprung's disease. *Upper trace,* rectosigmoid; *middle trace,* rectum; *lower trace,* anorectum

In our Diagnostic Work-up for Fecal Retention. Rectal manometry is carried out in all cases, regardless of whether abdominal X rays or radiographic contrast studies are necessary. If the internal sphincter relaxation reflex is normal, the patient is treated by conservative constipation therapy. If relaxation is absent or only rudimentary, mucosal biopsy is also performed for histology and histochemical acetylcholinesterase studies (Fig. 7). If ganglion cells are present, and acetylcholinesterase activity is low, myogenic achalasia can be diagnosed by further clinical examination (fibrous anal ring, cryptitis, fissure). Failure to demonstrate ganglion cells and increased acetylcholinesterase activity indicate aganglionosis. Hyperplasia of ganglion cells and of parasympathetic fibers point to neuronal intestinal dysplasia.

Evaluation of Continence. In order to evaluate continence, several manometric parameters must be examined. Incontinence is characterized by a pressure profile below 15 mm Hg (normal 25 mm Hg), an anorectal length of less than 2.5 cm (normal 3–5 cm), and usually an absent internal sphincter relaxation reflex. Squeeze pressure is less than 10 mm Hg (twice the normal resting pressure), and the duration of a voluntary contraction is less than 10 s (normal 30–50 s). Propulsive waves are not compensated by the anorectal muscles, and the adaptation reaction is generally lacking (Table 3; Schärli 1983). Intermediate measurements merely indicate partial continence. The same manometric also permit differentiation between neurogenic (meningomyelocele), myogenic (sphincter insufficiency), and constipation incontinence (overflow soiling) (Fig. 8).

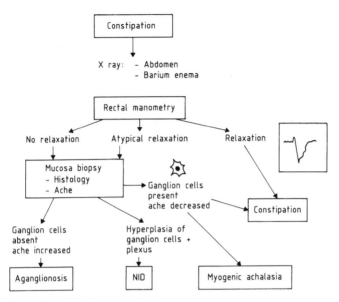

Fig. 7. Work-up for fecal retention

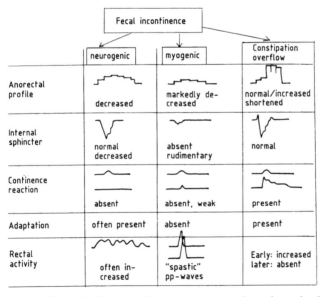

Fig. 8. Differential diagnosis of neurogenic, myogenic, and constipation incontinence

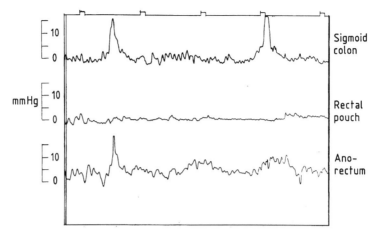

Fig. 9. Peristaltic activity absent in rectal blind pouch after Duhamel's operation. Anorectal conditions still pathological

- Neurogenic incontinence: The pressure profile is decreased; internal sphincter relaxation is normal or even low; no continence reaction is present. Rectal resting activity is often increased and the adaptation reaction preserved.
- Myogenic incontinence: There is a striking decrease in the anorectal pressure profile. Internal sphincter relaxation and the continence and adaptation reactions are also absent. Due to the lack of a sphincter barrier, propulsive waves are propagated directly through the anorectum.
- Constipation incontinence: The anorectal pressure profile is normal, but sphincter length is decreased. The relaxation reflex is maintained, as are continence and adaptation reactions. Rectal activity is increased early in the disorder but is absent in rectal inertia.

Manometric Studies in Postoperative Evaluation. As regards, first, megacolon surgery, we compared the results following Swenson's, Soave's, and Duhamel's procedures in 47 patients and determined that all three methods are capable of producing normal defecation and definitive cures (Schärli 1972). Postoperative internal sphincter relaxation appeared in five patients, which may be attributed to ingrowth of neural elements through the anastomosis. The manometric studies have also attracted attention to risks inherent in each operative procedure:

- If the anastomosis is too far away from the anorectal ring in Swenson's operation, there may be uncontrollable fecal congestion and a secondary megacolon.
- The risk in Soave's technique is high rectal stenosis due to shrinkage of the muscular rectal sheath.
- After Duhamel's procedure, we repeatedly observed that the residual rectal pouch does not participate in peristalsis: it is noncontracting, atonic, and enlarges progressively due to fecal accumulation (Fig. 9).

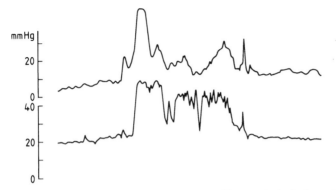

Fig. 10. Active contraction of musculus gracilis on arrival of a (perceived) propulsive wave. *Upper trace,* rectum; *lower trace,* anorectum

	Continence – Score	
	With/without drugs	With/without constipation
Normal		
Mucous staining		
Fecal soiling		
Incontinence		

0 Never; *1* rarely; *2* frequently; *3* continuously

Fig. 11. Evaluation of continence according to clinical parameters as proposed at Wingspread meeting, 1984

- After all methods, the internal sphincter may continue to react pathologically by contracting, making defecation extremely difficult or impossible. In these cases, partial posterior sphincterotomy is indicated.

Secondly, we have thus far performed manometric studies in 29 patients after gracilis transposition. This procedure elevates the anorectal pressure barrier and increases the capability for additional active contraction. In 18 cases, rectal adaptation with a clinical reservoir function appeared only after this operation. In all cases, the anorectal resting pressure profile decreased somewhat within several years. By active contraction, however, squeeze pressure was at least doubled in all patients, and maximal contractile force was constant for over 1 min (Fig. 10). All patients showed definite improvement on the Kelly clinical and manometric continence score. Critical analysis of all manometrically measureable components shows, however, that degree of continence cannot be analyzed by any one scoring system: decisive estimation of a patient's incontinence is purely clinical. The proposals from the 1984 Wingspread meeting, detailing four degrees of continence, appear to be a useful guideline (Wingspread Meeting 1984). Normal continence, mucous staining, fecal soiling, and fecal incontinence. It is also of significance whether these results are achieved with or without drugs and with or without constipation (Fig. 11).

Scientific Significance of Manometry

In addition to the constantly reproducible pressure changes in the anorectal profile during measurement of the squeeze pressure and internal sphincter relaxation, many measurements are dependent for interpretation on the particular experience of the examiner or may be scientifically analyzed. Among these are the adaptation reaction, studies of the induction of defecation and the propulsion process, and timed measurements of reflex propagation (Schärli and Kistler 1984). Our own studies have shown that the relaxation reflex is faster than normal in patients with chronic constipation, probably due to "thinning out" of the ganglion cells. In contrast, the speed of propagation is markedly diminished after surgery for megacolon.

It is also of scientific interest that a completely normal relaxation reflex can be demonstrated in the fistular zone of female patients with imperforate anus and rectovaginal fistula. This implies that the fistular tract actually corresponds to the embryonic anlage of the anorectum.

References

Arhan P, Faverdin C (1971) Technique d'exploration fonctionelle de la motricité digestive en chirurgie pédiatrique. Ann Chir Infant 12:197
Bayliss WM, Starling EH (1899) The movements and innervation of the small intestine. J Physiol (Lond) 24:99
Cannon WB (1939) A law of denervation. Am J Med Sci 198:737
Denny-Browne D, Robertson EG (1934) An investigation of the nervous control of defecation. Brain 57:256
Gowers WR (1877) The automatic action of the sphincter ani. Proc R Soc Med 26:77
Holschneider AM (1974) Differentialdiagnose und chirurgische Therapie der chronischen Obstipation im Kindesalter. Klin Padiatr 186:208
Holschneider AM, Metzler EM (1974) Manometrische Studien zur anorektalen Kontinenz im Kindesalter. Bruns Beitr Klin Chir 221:14
Holschneider AM, Keller E, Streibl P (1976) The development of anorectal continence and its significance for the diagnosis of Hirschsprung's disease. J Pediat Surg 11:151
Kelly JH (1972) The clinical and radiological assessment of anal continence in childhood. Aust N Z J Surg 42:62
Morikawa Y, Donahoe PK, Hendren WH (1979) Manometry and histochemistry in the diagnosis of Hirschsprung's disease. Pediatrics 63:865
Schärli AF (1971) Die angeborenen Missbildungen des Rektums und Anus. Huber, Bern
Schärli AF (1972) Funktionelle Untersuchungen beim Morbus Hirschsprung. Padiatr Pädol [Suppl] 2:32

Schärli AF (1982) The pathophysiology of Hirschsprung's disease. In: Holschneider AM (ed) Hirschsprung's disease. Hipokrates, Stuttgart

Schärli AF (1983) Analysis of anal incontinence. Prog Pediatr Surg 17

Schärli AF, Kiesewetter WB (1969) Anorectosigmoid pressure studies as a quantitative evaluation of continence. J Pediatr Surg 4:694

Schärli AF, Kiesewetter WB (1970) Defecation and continence: some new concepts. Dis Colon Rectum 13:81

Schärli AF, Kistler W (1984) Neue Aspekte über das Verhalten des Sphincter-internus-Relaxations-Reflexes. Z Kinderchir [Suppl I] 39:74–76

Schuster MM, Hookman P, Hendrix TR, Mendeloff AS (1965) Simultaneous manometric recording of internal and external anal sphincteric reflexes. Bull John Hopkins Hosp 116:79

Templeton RD, Lawson H (1932) Studies in motor activity of large intestine: response to autonomic drugs. Am J Physiol 101:511

Varma KK, Stephens D (1972) Neuromuscular reflexes of rectal continence. Aust N Z J Surg 41:263

Wingspread Meeting (1984) Meeting on the classification of anorectal anomalies. Racine, Wisconsin, March 25–27, 1984 (F.D. Stephens, E.D. Smith, organizers)

Functional Colonic Ultrasonography: Normal Findings of Colonic Motility and Follow-Up in Neuronal Intestinal Dysplasia

G. Pistor

Summary

Three types of neuronal intestinal dysplasia (type A, type B, and combination with Hirschsprung's disease) can be distinguished. Functional assessment of the affected bowel segments can be achieved by functional colonic ultrasonography, thus providing exact parameters for further therapeutical procedure. The technique is described. Ten children with neuronal intestinal dysplasia in whom functional colonic ultrasonography was employed and results of their follow-up examinations are reported.

Zusammenfassung

Drei Formen von neuronaler intestinaler Dysplasie (Typ A, Typ B, Kombination mit M. Hirschsprung) können unterschieden werden. Die funktionelle Beurteilung der betroffenen Darmabschnitte kann mit Hilfe der funktionellen Kolonsonographie erfolgen, die genaue Parameter für das weitere therapeutische Procedere liefert. Die Technik wird beschrieben. Es wird über 10 Kinder mit neuronaler intestinaler Dysplasie berichtet, bei denen die funktionelle Kolonsonographie auch zur Verlaufskontrolle eingesetzt wurde.

Résumé

On distingue trois formes de dysplasie intestinale neuronale (type A, type B, combinaison avec maladie de Hirschsprung). On évalue la fonction du segment intestinal atteint en pratiquant une échographie fonctionnelle du côlon qui fournira les paramètres précis pour poursuivre la thérapeutique. Cette technique est décrite. On rapporte le cas de plus de 10 enfants avec dysplasie intestinale neuronale, dont on suit l'évolution en utilisant l'échographie fonctionnelle du côlon.

Introduction

Radiography of the colon and endoscopy are standard methods in colonic diagnosis. Functional assessment of colonic motility by means of manometry (Cohen et al. 1968; Holschneider 1983; Nasmyth and Williams 1985) and electromyography (Quigley et al. 1984; Sarna et al. 1980) are chiefly of use for scientific problems rather than for clinical application. However, functional assessment of the affected bowel parts is of major importance for indication of colonic resection in neuronal

Pediatric Surgical Clinic, University of Mainz, Langenbeckstr. 1, D-6500 Mainz, FRG

intestinal dysplasia (NID) types A and B and in NID combined with Hirschsprung's disease since the course of the disease is predominantly influenced by changes in dysmotility of the large bowel.

NID type A is characterized by hypoplasia or aplasia of the sympathetic nervous system of the bowel wall. The disease starts early in most instances and shows an acute course. Characteristically, the major symptom is severe constipation, which may develop abruptly into ulcerous colitis. Found in 2% of cases of congenital dysganglionosis, the disease is rare (Meier-Ruge 1985). NID type B is much more common, occurring in 18% of innervation disturbances of the colon

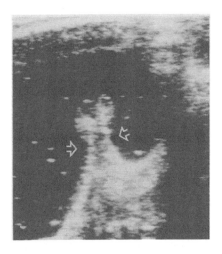

Fig. 1. Closed ileocecal valve. Sealing by marginal thickening. *Arrows*, closed vela

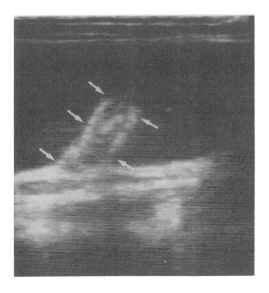

Fig. 2. Active opening of ileocecal valve by parallel branching of the vela *(arrows)*. Small amount of stools immediately in front of the valve

Functional Colonic Ultrasonography

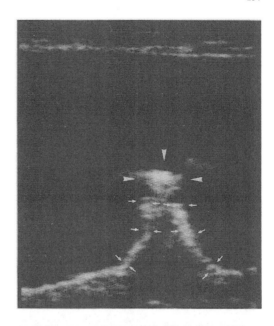

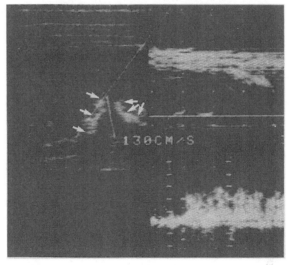

Fig. 3. a Passive opening of ileocecal valve by propulsive peristalsis of the terminal ileum. Injection of bowel contents into the cecum. **b** Measurement of flow speed during pressure-induced passive opening of ileocecal valve (jet phenomenon). Relatively high-flow speed and low-volume load of the cecum. *Arrows,* shape of valve at moment of bolus injection; *arrowheads,* injected bolus

(Meier-Ruge 1985). The disease is characterized by a hyperganglionosis of the submucous plexus. Development of a megacolon and predominantly chronic course are typical. Acute decompensation of NID-affected bowel segments is frequently observed in cases of NID combined with Hirschsprung's disease (Fadda et al. 1987). Functional maturation of the affected bowel is increasingly reported, thus avoiding early resection of the hyperganglionic bowel segments (Fadda et al.

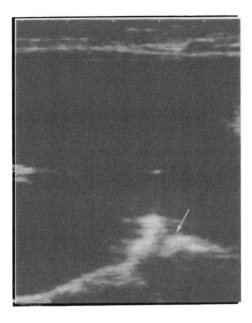

Fig. 4. Retrograde prolapse of the lower velum *(arrow)*

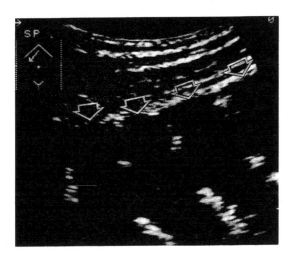

Fig. 5. Normal haustration, lumen width, and wall thickness of the ascending colon. *Arrows,* anterior wall of ascending colon

1983, 1987; Meier-Ruge 1985; Munakata et al. 1985; Pistor et al. 1984, 1987a, b; Sacher et al. 1982). Clinical parameters alone are insufficient or uncertain for the assessment of improvement in motility in NID since a colostomy has often been established to relieve the bowel. Therefore, functional colonic ultrasonography is employed for functional assessment (Pistor et al. 1984).

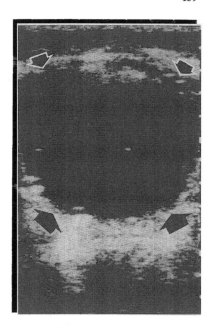

Fig. 6. Megarectum with cross-section *(arrows)* of 9 cm in an 8-year-old body

Material and Methods

The technique of functional colonic ultrasonography is as follows. The colon is irrigated by 20–50 ml/kg body weight Ringer's solution heated to 30°C transanally or via colostomy by means of a blocked-bladder catheter. When a filling pressure of 20 cm H_2O has been reached, the whole colon is morphologically assessed. Functional investigation by means of a high-resolution 5-MHz real-time scanner starts 10 min after pressure stabilization and is continuously recorded on magnetic tape.

From 1981 to 1986, 200 infants and children of all age groups were examined by this method, among them ten patients with NID. The following functional and morphological parameters were investigated ultrasonographically and compared with normal findings:

1. Motility and morphology of the ileocecal region and passive and active function of the ileocecal valve (Pistor et al. 1987a, b; Figs. 1–4).

2. Morphological assessment of colonic haustration (Fig. 5), width of lumen (Fig. 6), and wall thickness (Fig. 7).

3. Colonic motility with assessment of concentric wall contractions (Fig. 8), haustral contractions, mass contractions (Fig. 9), shortening (Fig. 10), segmentation (Fig. 11), rectal motility, and transverse folds of the rectum (Kohlrausch's fold; Figs. 12, 13).

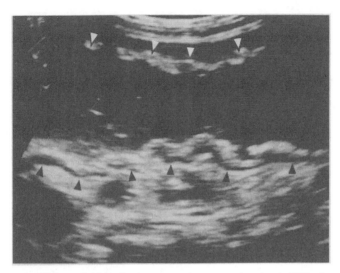

Fig. 7. Slight wall thickening in a regressing megacolon due to NID. *Arrows,* thickened and wary wall of colon

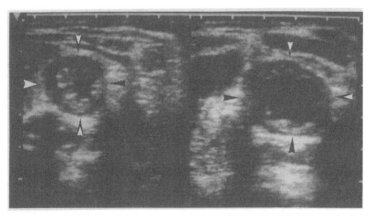

Fig. 8. Concentric contraction. Cross-section *(arrows)* at the left flexure. *Left,* contraction; *right,* advanced contraction

Results

Colonic motility of the affected bowel segments was examined in ten children with NID by means of functional colonic ultrasonography. Four children did not exhibit functional disturbances of the hyperganglionic segments during a follow-up period of 3 years, but the first ultrasonographic examination revealed hypomotile disturbances of the large intestine in six children (Figs. 7, 10). Four of these

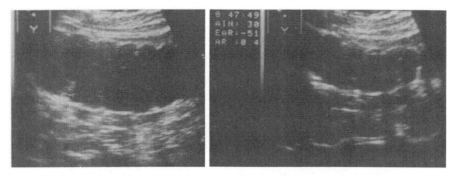

Fig. 9. Propulsive mass contractions from descending to the sigmoid colon. *Left,* beginning contraction; *right,* advanced contraction

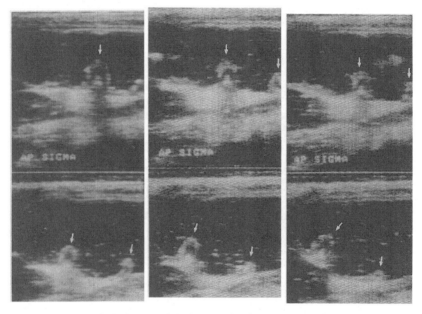

Fig. 10. Shortening by pathological haustra in NID. *Arrows,* the haustrum is displaced proximally by longitudinal contraction of the transverse colon (no haustral flowing)

six children achieved nearly complete normalization of peristalsis during a follow-up period of up to 3.5 years after establishment of colostomy. No change of distal colonic adynamia was seen in an 8-year-old boy. In this boy the resection plane was established by means of functional ultrasonographic parameters. Another patient was only recently investigated. Normal motion patterns of the ileocecel region were seen in all patients.

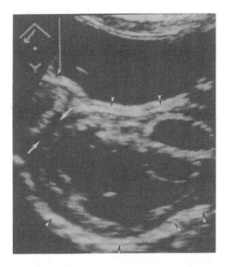

Fig. 11. Rectal segmentation. *Arrows,* segmentations due to Kohlrausch's fold; *arrowheads,* anterior and posterior walls of rectum

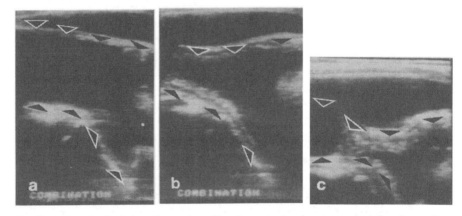

Fig. 12a–c. Longitudinal view of megasigmoid and megarectum in compensated chronic constipation. **a** Distended rectum. *Arrows,* anterior and posterior walls. **b** Propulsive contraction. *Arrows,* walls of half-contracted rectum. **c** Complete contraction and segmentation of Kohlrausch's fold *(arrows)*

Discussion

Improved diagnosis of colonic motility disturbances in recent years has increased the rate of diagnosed NID cases (Fadda et al. 1983, 1987; Meier-Ruge 1985; Munakata et al. 1985; Pistor et al. 1987a, b). The disease appears in three forms: (a) isolated type A, (b) isolated type B, and (c) combined with Hirschsprung's disease (Fadda et al. 1988). Histologically and histochemically, type A is characterized by hypoplasia and aplasia, respectively, of the sympathetic nervous system. In type B a hyperganglionosis of the submucous plexus is found (Meier-Ruge

Functional Colonic Ultrasonography

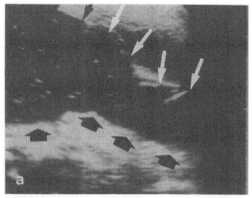

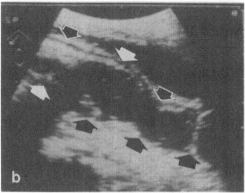

Fig. 13a, b. Combined NID and Hirschsprung's disease. **a** Transition zone from slight hyperganglionic colonic distention via short funnel into narrow aganglionic segment. **b** Normal propulsive contraction in hyperganglionic segment and cessation of peristaltic wave at beginning of aganglionic segment. *White arrows* mark ventral wall of transition zone and aganglionic segment

1985). The rare type A participates in 3% of cases of Hirschsprung's disease (Meier-Ruge 1985), whereas the incidence of type B and the combination with Hirschsprung's disease differ hardly from each other, with an incidence that is one-fourth to one-third of that of Hirschsprung's disease. The increased incidence of combined NID and Hirschsprung's disease in recent years can be attributed to a more careful diagnosis of suspicious Hirschsprung cases (Fadda et al. 1987). The acute early signs of type A and combined NID and Hirschsprung's disease can hardly be differentiated by clinical findings (Fadda et al. 1987). Type B most commonly shows a chronic course, with pronounced colonic hypomotility and development of a megacolon (Meier-Ruge 1985). The extent of histological-histochemical changes, however, does not correlate either with the severity of disease (Fadda et al. 1983) or with colonic dysmotility as major symptom. Despite persistent morphological changes, functional maturation of NID has been reported in type B (Munakata et al. 1985; Pistor et al. 1984, 1987a, b) as well as in combination with Hirschsprung's disease (Fadda et al. 1983).

Problems, however, arise from the timing of colostomy and colon resection if clinical parameters alone are referred to since sufficient defecation from the colostomy is possible also in an affected bowel, with persistent dysmotility due to the low opening pressure of the colostomy. Colostomy or bowel resection performed too early or insufficiently may cause renewed decompensation of hyperganglionic segments due to elevated pressure, if maturation does not occur or has not yet taken place.

We were able to find persistent colonic motility disturbances by means of functional colonic ultrasonography in four children who had obviously normal defecation via colostomy. Repeated follow-up examinations over years showed nearly complete functional maturation. Improvement of colonic motility could be demonstrated up to the 4th year of life. Another four children with combined NID and Hirschsprung's disease did not present with functional disturbances of the hyperganglionic segments. None of these children developed postoperative complications due to renewed motility disorders following resection of the aganglionic segments where the hyperganglionic segments were left in place. Children in whom colonic motility disturbances of hyperganglionic segments persist beyond the 4th year of life should not have further conservative treatment since improvement of peristalsis can no longer be awaited. In this case it is recommended to determine the extent of resection of the diseased bowel by means of functional ultrasonography. Experiences over recent years have shown that resection up to the left flexure is generally sufficient, even if NID was proven more proximal by histological examination.

References

Cohen S, Harris LD, Levitan R (1968) Manometric characteristics of the human ileocecal junctional zone. Gastroenterology 54:72–75

Fadda B, Maier WA, Meier-Ruge W, Schärli A, Daum R (1983) Neuronale intestinale Dysplasie. Z Kinderchir 38(5):305–311

Fadda B, Pistor G, Meier-Ruge W, Hofmann-von Kap-herr S, Müntefering H, Espinoza R (1987) Symptoms, diagnosis and therapy of neuronal intestinal dysplasia masked by Hirschsprung's disease. Report of 24 cases. Pediatr Surg Int 2:76–80

Holschneider AM (1983) Elektromanometrie des Enddarms, 2nd edn. Urban and Schwarzenberg, Munich

Meier-Ruge W (1985) Angeborene Dysganglionosen des Colons. Kinderarzt 16(2):151–164

Munakata K, Morita K, Okabe J, Sueoka H (1985) Clinical and histologic studies of neuronal intestinal dysplasie. J Pediatr Surg 20(3):231–235

Nasmyth DG, Williams NS (1985) Pressure characteristics of the human ileocecal region – a key to its function. Gastroenterology 345–351

Pistor G, Hofmann-von Kap-herr S (1984) Funktionelle Colonsonographie bei neuronaler intestinaler Dysplasie – Bericht über drei Fälle. Fortschr Med 102(14):397–400

Pistor G, Hofmann- von Kap-herr S, Grüssner R, Munakata K, Müntefering H (1987a) Neuronal intestinal dysplasia. Modern diagnosis and therapy, report of 23 patients. Pediatr Surg Int 2:352–358

Pistor G, Eckmann A, Grüssner R, Weltzien A (1987b) Funktionelle Echomorphologie der Bauhin'schen Klappe. Fortschr Roentgenstr 146,3:278–283

Quigley EMM, Borody TJ, Phillips SF, Wienbeck M, Tucker RL, Haddad A (1984) Motility of the terminal ileum and ileocecal sphincter in healthy humans. Gastroenterology 87:857–866

Sacher P, Briner U, Stauffer UG (1982) Zur klinischen Bedeutung der neuronalen intestinalen Dysplasie. Z Kinderchir 35:96–97

Sarna SK, Bardakjian BL, Waterfall WE, Lind JF (1980) Human colonic electrical control activity (ECA). Gastroenterology 78:1526–1536

The Influence of Small Bowel Contamination on the Pathogenesis of Bowel Obstruction

M. Schwöbel[1], J. Hirsig[1], O. Illi[1], and U. Bättig[2]

Summary

Altered motility of the intestine after laparotomy, adynamic bowel segments, blind bowel loops following bypass operations, or diverticula may cause pathological growth of intestinal microflora and thus lead to contaminated small bowel syndrome (CSBS). As a result of malabsorption in the jejunum and ileum, loss of weight, growth arrest, diarrhea, steatorrhea, megaloblastic anemia, and hypoproteinemia may occur. In addition to these, the acute symptoms of small bowel contamination, intestinal obstruction and secretory diarrhea, are less well known.

A stenosis in the terminal ileum was experimentally created in Göttingen minipigs and the bacterial flora of the small bowel assessed by quantitative cultures. After 3 months the number of aerobic and anaerobic bacteria in the pre- and poststenotic region had increased by a factor of 10^2–10^5.

The acute form of CSBS was diagnosed by microbiological examination of gastric samples in 14 children. After the children were treated with orally and intravenously administered antibiotics, the symptoms disappeared within 12–36 h. Reoperations for small bowel obstruction can be avoided by conservative treatment of CSBS with antibiotics.

Zusammenfassung

Postoperative Störungen der Darmmotilität, adyname Darmabschnitte, blinde Schlingen nach Bypassoperationen oder Divertikel können eine pathologische Vermehrung der intestinalen Mikroflora verursachen und damit zum Syndrom des kontaminierten Dünndarms führen. Als Folge einer Malabsorption in Jejunum und Ileum kommt es dabei zu Gewichtsabnahme, Wachstumsstillstand, Durchfällen, Steatorrhö, megaloblastärer Anämie und Hypoproteinämie. Weniger bekannt sind die akuten Folgen der Dünndarmkontamination, nämlich Ileus und sekretorische Diarrhö. Bei Göttinger Minipigs wurde experimentell eine Stenose im Bereich des terminalen Ileums gebildet und die Bakterienzahl pro Milliliter in regelmäßigen Abständen gemessen. Nach 3 Monaten war die Menge aerober und anaerober Bakterien prä- und poststenotisch um einen Faktor zwischen 10^2 und 10^5 angestiegen.

Bei 14 Kindern mit der akuten Form des Syndroms wurde die Diagnose aus der Magensaftbakteriologie gestellt. Anschließend wurden die Kinder mit peroral und intravenös verabreichten Antibiotika behandelt. Die Ileussymptome verschwanden innerhalb 12–36 h. Wird das Syndrom des kontaminierten Dünndarms gezielt antibiotisch behandelt, können Reoperationen wegen Motilitätsstörungen des Dünndarms vermieden werden.

Résumé

Les troubles de la motilité intestinale post-opératoire, les segments adynamiques de l'intestin, les anses borgnes après opération de pontage et les diverticules peuvent amener une pullulation

---

[1] Pediatric Surgical Clinic, University Children's Hospital, Steinwiesstr. 75, CH-8032 Zurich
[2] Institute of Veterinary Bacteriology, University of Zurich, Winterthurer Str. 270, CH-8032 Zurich, Switzerland

microbienne et conduire ainsi au syndrome de l'anse borgne. Les troubles de l'absorption qui vont s'en suivre au niveau du jéjunum et de l'iléon amèneront des diarrhées, une stéatorrhée, une anémie mégaloblastique, une hypoprotéinémie avec enfin une perte de poids et un arrêt de croissance. Les conséquences immédiates d'une contamination de l'intestin grêle, à savoir iléus et diarrhées inflammatoires, sont moins connues. Expérimentalement fut réalisée sur des minipigs de Göttingen une sténose au niveau de l'iléon terminal; le nombre de bactéries par ml a été ensuite mesuré à intervalles réguliers. Après trois mois la quantité de bactéries aérobes et anaérobes prélevées dans la région pré- et poststénotique s'est multipliée par un facteur de 10^2 à 10^5. Chez 14 enfants présentant une forme aiguë de ce syndrome, le diagnostic a été établi par l'examen bactériologique du suc gastrique. Une antibiothérapie orale et intraveineuse a amené la disparition des symptomes d'occlusion en l'espace de 12 à 36 heures.

Un traitement antibiotique approprié devrait permettre d'éviter une chirurgie itérative pour trouble de la motilité de l'intestin grêle.

Introduction

The microflora of the human gastrointestinal tract represents a highly complex ecosystem. Pathological changes in the composition of the bacterial population may lead to the contaminated small bowel syndrome (CSBS). As a consequence of malabsorption in the jejunum and ileum, arrest of growth or weight loss, diarrhea, steatorrhea, megaloblastic anemia, and hypoproteinemia may result. The acute symptoms of CSBS, small bowel obstruction and secretory diarrhea are described in the present paper.

Case Reports

K. M. This girl was born with a type III esophageal atresia, duodenal atresia and anal atresia with anovestibular fistula. The malformations were operated in the neonatal period. Due to anastomotic leakage in the esophagus, a cervical esophageal fistula was established and secondary esophageal replacement by means of the transverse colon was later carried out. Despite her severe malformations the girl developed well. Her weight was slight below the 3rd percentile; her size was between the 3rd and 10th percentile.

At the age of 7.5 years, she was admitted to our hospital for colicky abdominal pain lasting for 24 h and stool retention accompanied by bile-stained vomiting for 12 h. On physical examination, the abdomen was distended but soft. The lower abdomen was sensitive to pressure and tapping. Bowel sounds were increased and metallic. Plain abdominal X ray revealed multiple fluid levels, thus leading to the diagnosis of mechanical bowel obstruction. As first measure a nasogastric tube was inserted into the stomach, and bacteriological examination of gastric juice was performed. Gram staining revealed numerous gram-negative organisms; *Escherichia coli, Neisseria,* and *Clostridium* were found in microbial culture. Therapy with co-trimoxazole and ornidazole, simultaneously administered intravenously and via nasogastric tube, was initiated. The nasogastric tube could be withdrawn after 24 h, and the girl was fed orally without problems. Follow-up has now been for 4 years. No further hospitalization has been necessary. The girl takes anti-

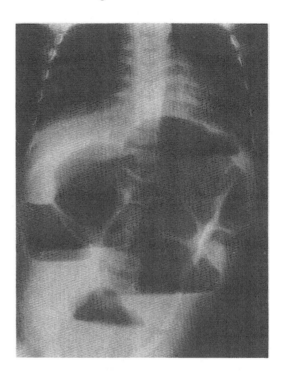

Fig. 1. Patient G.P. A 5.5-month-old, small-bowel obstruction. Note the grossly distended bowel loops and multiple fluid levels

biotics perorally for a few days once a month and feels well. Her weight is now at the 3rd percentile.

G. P. In this boy with EMG syndrome (exomphalos, macroglossia, gigantism) an omphalocele was closed on the 1st day of life. He had to undergo relaparotomy for small-bowel volvulus at the age of 5 weeks, and only 60 cm of small bowel could be left in place. Following three further relaparotomies, a side-to-side anastomosis between the remaining terminal ileum and the colon was performed. During the following months the boy developed profuse diarrhea and bile-stained vomiting. Plain abdominal X-ray revealed distended bowel loops and multiple fluid levels (Fig. 1). Bacteriological examination of gastric juice showed growth of *E. coli,* Klebsiellae, and anaerobic germs. Therefore, continuous therapy with co-trimoxazol and ornidazole was initiated, leading to rapid improvement of the child. His weight increased to over the 50th percentile (Fig. 2), and stool frequency declined to two or three defecations per day. Since then over 3 years have passed and no further hospitalization has become necessary.

B. G. This 13-year-old boy was operated for acute appendicitis ante perforationem. An abdominal drainage tube was not inserted. He was given co-trimoxazole and ornidazole postoperatively. During the following 48 h, the boy developed bowel obstruction, necessitating relaparotomy. Massively dilated bowel loops were

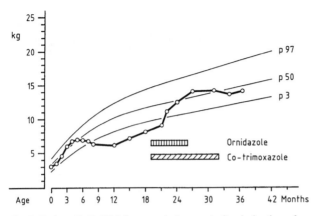

Fig. 2. Patient G. P. Weight curve before and after induction of peroral chemotherapy

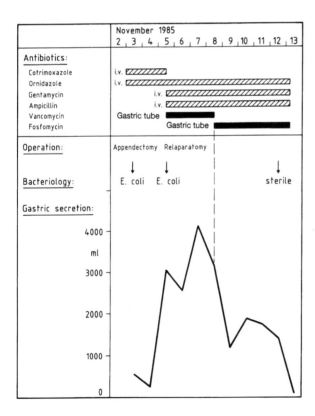

Fig. 3. Patient B.G. Schema of course, treatment, bacteriology, and gastric juice analysis in a 13-year-old boy

seen, but neither stump leakage nor a mechanical cause for bowel obstruction could be found. Intraoperatively 4 l of bowel contents were aspirated. The boy's clinical condition did not improve postoperatively. More than 4 l gastric juice per day were drained via a nasogastric tube. *E. coli*, not sensitive to cotrimoxazole was cultured after both operations. After administration of fosfomycin via a jejunal catheter the boy's condition improved rapidly (Fig. 3). Secretion of gastric juice decreased, and the nasogastric tube could be withdrawn within 2 days.

Discussion

The neonatal gastrointestinal tract is populated by aerobic and anaerobic bacteria in an oral-aboral direction (Bishop and Anderson 1960; Challacombe et al. 1974). In the fasting individual the typical gastric flora consists of few gram-positive bacteria and acid-resistant germs (Challacombe et al. 1974; Simon and Gorbach 1984). Enterobacteriae may be present in small amounts; anaerobic germs are missing. The duodenal and jejunal microflora corresponds to that of the stomach (Thadepalli et al. 1979). More aborally, Enterococci, *E. coli*, Klebsiellae, and anaerobic germs are found in increasing numbers (Nichols et al. 1971). Distal to the ileocecal valve, bacterial concentrations increase sharply.

We speak of contamination if Enterobacteriae, Enterococci, and anaerobic germs are abundant (10^6 germs/ml) in stomach, jejunum, and proximal ileum. Pathological bacterial growth proximal to the obstruction, including duodenum and stomach, is found in newborns with total small-bowel obstruction. The bowel distal to the obstruction remains sterile. In stenoses, however, contamination takes place also distal to the obstruction (Bishop and Anderson 1960). The diagnosis of CSBS is of complex nature and is based either on direct aspiration of jejunal juice or on indirect indicators such as deconjugation of bile acids by anaerobic bacteria (Haan et al. 1985; King et al. 1979). Bishop and Anderson (1960) found in 19 children with small-bowel obstruction, gastric juice contaminated with *E. coli* in 15 instances. Since our own experiences (Schwöbel et al. 1985) confirm these findings, we have made the diagnosis of CSBS by means of microscopic (gram-staining) and bacteriological examination of the gastric juice in children with bowel obstruction.

Chronic CSBS leads to weight loss, steatorrhea, megaloblastic anemia, and hypoproteinemia (Drenick et al. 1976; Gracey 1979; Haan et al. 1985; King and Toskes 1979; McEvoy et al. 1983; Savino 1982; Stern and Lambrecht 1982). It is assumed that bile acids deconjugated by anaerobic bacteria as well as bacterial toxins influence the mucosa directly, thus causing malabsorption in the jejunum and ileum. In rats with self-filling disconnected small-bowel loops Menge et al. (1985) have shown the overgrowth of *E. coli*, Enterococci and anaerobic germs by bacteriological examination and the damage of the mucosa by light and electron microscopy.

The acute form of CSBS may lead to secretory diarrhea and ileus. Toxinogenic bacteria *(E. coli, Shigella dysenteriae, Vibrio cholerae)* influence, possibly by acti-

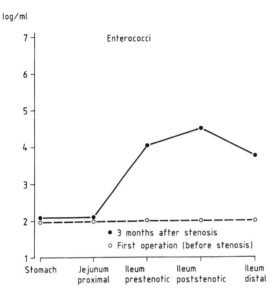

Fig. 4. Number of enterococci per milliliter aspirated juice before and 3 months following experimental production of a small-bowel stenosis

vation of the adenyl cyclase, the balance between secretion and absorption of water and electrolytes in villi and crypts in favor of secretion. Enterotoxins cause a reversible functional defect of mucosal cells (Banwell 1975; Hendrix 1975). Active secretion of bowel mucosa starts 15–30 min following the exposition of a bowel sling to enterotoxin, achieving a maximum after 10–18 h. Infants and children are more sensitive than adults. Fluid accumulation is an effect of the local bacterial population. Heneghan et al. (1981) have shown in dogs raised in a sterile milieu that the bowel sling proximal to an obstruction absorbs fluid, whereas in dogs raised in a normal environment the bowel flora provokes secretion which leads to accumulation of fluid. An animal model for the acute form of CSBS has not yet been established. We have tried in Göttingen mini-pigs (Beglinger et al. 1975) to provoke a contamination by surgically obstructing the ileum. Whereas the number of aerobic and anaerobic bacteria increased in the bowel lumen postoperatively (Fig. 4), no animal developed diarrhea or vomiting. Further experiments with extreme stenoses and sham-operated control animals will show whether a significant bacterial contamination of the pig bowel can be produced experimentally.

The acute form of CSBS starts with motility disturbances of the bowel. The balance of intestinal microflora was altered by stasis in the colon serving for esophageal replacement in our first patient, missing ileocecal valve, a blind-ending pouch and a long side-to-side anastomosis between the small and large bowel in our patient with short bowel syndrome, and postoperative bowel paralysis in our appendectomized patient. Bile acids deconjugated by anaerobic bacteria and enterotoxins damaged the mucosa, resulting in massive secretion of water and electrolytes into the bowel lumen. Massively fluid-filled bowel slings kinked proximal to a relative stenosis, thus leading to total stenosis and the clinical picture of mechanical bowel obstruction. Reoperations may not be useful in these situations. However, if the overgrowing bacteria are treated directly by antibiotics, obstructive symptoms may disappear within 12-36 h.

If small-bowel contamination is suspected, the following procedure proves efficacious: sampling of gastric or jejunal juice via appropriate tube, gram staining and bacteriological culture, and treatment of aerobic and anaerobic bacteria by simultaneous intravenous and enteral administration of antibiotics. Combination of co-trimoxazole and ornidazole have been shown to be useful. If gram-positive cocci are found abundantly, ornidazole is replaced by vancomycin. The patients are clinically examined at short intervals after conservative treatment has begun. Prerequisites of conservative treatment are absence of peritonitic signs and improvement of symptoms within 12-24 h. During the past 30 months, we have treated 14 children with ileus by this procedure, we feel that antimicrobial treatment of CSBS may help to avoid reoperations for small-bowel obstruction.

References

Banwell JG (1975) The influence of *Escherichia coli* and other bacterial enterotoxins on intestinal fluid transport. In: Csaky TZ (ed) Intestinal absorption and malabsorption. Raven, New York, pp 273-284
Beglinger R, Becker M, Eggenberger E, Lombard C (1975) Das Göttinger Miniaturschwein als Versuchstier. 1. Mitteilung: Literaturübersicht, Zucht und Haltung, Kreislaufparameter. Res Exp Med (Berl) 165:251-263
Bishop RF, Anderson CM (1960) The bacterial flora of the stomach and small intestine in children with intestinal obstruction. Arch Dis Child 35:487-491
Challacombe DN, Richardson JM, Anderson CM (1974) Bacterial microflora of the upper gastrointestinal tract in infants without diarrhoea. Arch Dis Child 49:264-269
Drenick EJ, Ament ME, Finegold SM, Passaro E (1976) Bypass enteropathy. Intestinal and systemic manifestations following small bowel bypass. JAMA 236:269-272
Gracey M (1979) The contaminated small bowel syndrome: pathogenesis, diagnosis and treatment. Am J Clin Nutr 32:234-243
Haan E, Brown G, Bankier A, Mitchell D, Hunt S, Blakey J, Barnes G (1985) Severe illness caused by the products of bacterial metabolism in a child with a short gut. Eur J Pediatr 144: 63-65
Hendrix TR (1975) Cholera toxin and intestinal transport. In: Csaky TZ (ed) Intestinal absorption and malabsorption. Raven, New York, pp 253-271
Heneghan JB, Robinson JWL, Menge H, Winistörfer B (1981) Intestinal obstruction in germfree dogs. Eur J Clin Invest 11:285-290
King CE, Toskes PP (1979) Small intestine bacterial overgrowth. Gastroenterology 76:1035-1055
King CE, Toskes PP, Spivey JC, Lorenz E, Welkos S (1979) Detection of small intestine bacterial overgrowth by means of a ^{14}C-D-xylose breath test. Gastroenterology 77:75-82
McEvoy A, Dutton J, James OFW (1983) Bacterial contamination of the small intestine is an important cause of occult malabsorption in the elderly. Br Med J 287:789
Menge H, Germer CT, Stössel R, Simes G, Wagner J, Hahn H, Riecken ED (1985) Untersuchungen zur Bedeutung der bakteriellen Fehlbesiedelung in der Pathogenese der Schleimhautschädigung beim experimentellen Blindsacksyndrom. Schweiz Med Wochenschr 115: 1012-1013

Nichols RL, Condon RE, Bentley DW, Gorbach SL (1971) Ileal microflora in surgical patients. J Urol 105:351–353
Savino JA (1982) Malabsorption secondary to Meckel's diverticulum. Am J Surg 144:588–592
Schwöbel M, Hirsig J, Stauffer UG (1985) Die Kontamination des Dünndarms als Ursache von Ileusepisoden beim darmoperierten Kind. Z Kinderchir 40:228–232
Simon GL, Gorbach SL (1984) Intestinal flora in health and disease. Gastroenterology 86:174–193
Stern M, Lambrecht W (1982) Meckel'sches Divertikel and Syndrom der blinden Schlinge. Monatsschr Kinderheilkd 130:165–167
Thadepalli H, Lou MA, Bach VT, Matsui TK, Mandal AK (1979) Microflora of the human small intestine. Am J Surg 138:845–850

Diagnosis of Innervation-Related Motility Disorders of the Gut and Basic Aspects of Enteric Nervous System Development

J. C. Molenaar[1], D. Tibboel[1], A. W. M. van der Kamp[2], and J. H. C. Meijers[1]

Summary

Motility disorders of the gut in children have become a matter of increasing concern for the pediatric surgeon. Infantile hypertrophic pyloric stenosis is the most common disease requiring surgery in early infancy. While this entity was first described as early as 1888 by Hirschsprung, its etiology and pathogenesis are still an enigma. Fortunately, its surgical treatment is simple and safe, which cannot be said of all other motility disorders of the infantile gut.

Dysmotility in small bowel atresia and in gastroschisis is related to damaged smooth muscle cells caused by concomitant ischemia of the bowel wall. In contrast, the temporarily adynamic bowel of the prematurely born child, as well as Hirschsprung's disease and related disorders, is the result of anomalies of the intestinal innervation. The pathogenesis of congenital malformations of the enteric nervous system is still a mystery to surgeons and physicians alike.

With his pressure studies of the colon, Swenson first recognized Hirschsprung's disease for what it was. This led to the resection of the manometrically diagnosed abnormal colon, which was found to be aganglionic. Histological investigation of the bowel wall became the decisive tool, replacing manometry, in the diagnosis of Hirschsprung's disease. Histochemical investigation of the bowel wall is not conclusive in other malformations of the enteric nervous system, since the presence or absence of enteric neurons is not the definitive factor discriminating between normally and abnormally functioning bowel. Monoclonal antibodies raised against neuron-specific markers may become important tools for differentiation within the spectrum of congenital malformations of the enteric nervous system. The immunocytochemical technique, however, does not provide sufficient information to explain the cause of innervation disorders of the gut in infancy and childhood.

Primary migration disturbances or selective disappearance of enteric neurons following ischemia are highly unlikely to cause aganglionosis of the gut. With respect to the pathogenesis and etiology of Hirschsprung's disease, current research is focused on the embryonic bowel (target organ) in plexus formation.

The enteric nervous system is still an enigma, although its origin is known, at least in birds. Why neural crest cells travel, along what paths, how they reach their destination, and what may go wrong during the migratory process, are questions that must be answered. There is increasing knowledge concerning the way in which neural crest cells aggregate and form plexuses in the gut. It is largely unknown why neural crest cells settle, in the bowel, at the sites of the myenteric and submucous plexus. Ongoing developmental biological research and detailed neuropathological characterization of congenital malformations of the enteric nervous system will lead to a better understanding of the pathogenesis and, consequently, a proper treatment and prevention of these congenital malformations.

---

[1]Department of Pediatric Surgery, [2]Department of Cell Biology and Genetics, Erasmus University School of Medicine, Sophia Children's Hospital, P. O. Box 70029, 3000 LL Rotterdam, The Netherlands

Zusammenfassung

Motilitätsstörungen des Darmes im Kindesalter erhalten zunehmende Bedeutung für den Kinderchirurgen. Die infantile hypertrophische Pylorusstenose ist die häufigste Erkrankung, die einer chirurgischen Intervention im frühen Säuglingsalter bedarf. Während dieses Krankheitsbild bereits im Jahre 1888 von Harold Hirschsprung beschrieben wurde, bleiben Ätiologie und Pathogenese auch heute noch ein Rätsel. Glücklicherweise ist die chirurgische Behandlung einfach und sicher, was man nicht von allen anderen Motilitätsstörungen des kindlichen Darmes sagen kann.

Die Dünndarmdysmotilität bei der Dünndarmatresie und der Gastroschisis hat mit Innervationsstörungen nichts zu tun, sondern ist ausschließlich das Produkt einer Schädigung der Darmmuskulatur durch begleitende Darmwandischämie. Hingegen sind die temporäre Darmadynamie des Frühgeborenen sowie der M. Hirschsprung mit seinen Begleiterscheinungen das Resultat abnormer Darminnervation. Obwohl die Aganglionie schon seit langem als kongenitale Fehlbildung erkannt worden ist, bleibt die neuronale Dysplasie (abnorme Gewebeentwicklung) für Chirurgen und Internisten gleichermaßen auch heute noch ungeklärt.

Swenson klärte als erster mit seinen Druckuntersuchungen des Kolons die Natur des M. Hirschsprung. Daraufhin wurde die Resektion des durch Manometrie als abnorm erkannten Kolons, das aganglionär ist, eingeführt. Die histologische Untersuchung der Darmwand wurde dann die entscheidende Untersuchungsmethode beim M. Hirschsprung, die die Manometrie ersetzte. Ihre Verläßlichkeit wird jedoch wieder angezweifelt, da der Befund einer Ganglionose oder Aganglionose letztlich nicht der entscheidende Faktor ist, durch den normal und abnorm innervierter Darm unterschieden werden kann. Ebensowenig liefert sie genügend Information, um alle Ursachen der Darminnervationsstörungen im Säuglings- und Kindesalter zu klären. Viele Hypothesen wurden aufgestellt.

Das enterische Nervensystem gibt immer noch Rätsel auf, obwohl dessen Herkunft zumindest bei Vögeln bekannt ist. Warum Neuralleistenzellen wandern, welche Wege sie nehmen, wie sie ihren Bestimmungort erreichen und was bei diesem Migrationsprozeß fehlerhaft ablaufen kann, dies alles sind offene Fragen, die beantwortet werden müssen, bevor die volle Aufklärung und somit eine effektive Behandlung der neuronalen Dysplasie erreicht werden kann.

Résumé

Les troubles de la motilité intestinale chez les enfants prennent de plus en plus d'importance pour le chirurgien pédiatrique. La sténose du pylore hypertrophique infantile est l'affection la plus fréquente et requiert une intervention chirurgicale dans la période néonatale. Cette affection a été décrite dès 1888 par Harold Hirschsprung mais son étiologie et sa pathogénie n'ont pas encore été élucidées. Heureusement, le traitement chirurgical est simple et sans risques, ce qui n'est pas le cas des autres formes de troubles de la motilité de l'intestin dans l'enfance.

La dysmotilité de l'intestin grêle dans les cas d'atrésie de celui-ci et de laparoschisis n'est pas du tout liée à des troubles de l'innervation mais est due exclusivement à une lésion de la musculature intestinale causée par une ischémie concomitante de la paroi intestinale. Par contre, l'adynamie intestinale temporaire et la maladie de Hirschsprung et ses manifestations secondaires sont bien le résultat d'une innervation anormale de l'intestin. Bien que l'on sache depuis longtemps que l'aganglionie constitue une malformation congénitale, la dysplasie neuronale reste un mystère pour les chirurgiens et les internistes. C'est Swenson qui, le premier, fit la lumière sur la nature de la maladie de Hirschsprung en mesurant la pression du côlon. On introduisit alors la résection du côlon que la manométrie avait révélé anormal puisqu'aganglionnaire. L'examen histologique de la paroi intestinale devint alors l'examen de choix dans le cas de la maladie de Hirschsprung et remplaça la manométrie. On commence entretemps à émettre des doutes sur sa fiabilité, étant donné qu'une ganglionose ou une aganglionose n'est pas l'élément essentiel permettant de distinguer une innervation normale d'une innervation anormale de l'intestin. Cet examen ne fournit en outre pas assez d'informations pour faire la lumière sur toutes les causes des troubles de l'innervation de l'intestin chez les nouveaux-nés et les enfants. Plusieurs hypothèses ont été avancées.

Le système nerveux entérique pose encore bien des énigmes bien que ses origines soient connues, du moins chez les oiseaux. Pourquoi les cellules des crêtes neuronales se déplacent-elles, quelles voies empruntent-elles, comment parviennent-elles à leur destination et quelles pannes peuvent se produire durant cette migration, autant de questions auxquelles il va falloir apporter une réponse avant d'être en possession de tous les éléments permettant un traitement efficace des dysplasies neuronales.

Introduction

The food we eat must be processed for absorption. Consequently, any malfunction or obstruction of the digestive tract is potentially life threatening. The absorption of food is totally dependent on the propulsive motility and free passage of our digestive tract. Normal propulsive motility is totally dependent on a normal musculature and normal innervation of the intestinal wall. The musculature forms a continuous, uninterrupted structure from the upper part of the esophagus to the anus. Sphincters are functional rather than anatomical entities.

Extrinsic and intrinsic nerves, with afferent and efferent pathways, control the excitatory and inhibitory input of the smooth muscle cells. The "enteric nervous system," a really smart system, functions like a second "brain" and coordinates and programs all gastrointestinal functions. A myriad of chemoreceptors and mechanoreceptors located in the intestinal wall detect the presence and volume of food and its chemical properties. Unfortunately, this system is so deeply embedded in the gut wall that it is practically inaccessible for investigation or experimentation. This has hampered the diagnosis and pharmaceutical management of many motility disorders.

Motility disorders in children have assumed increasing importance for the pediatric gastroenterologist as well as for the pediatric surgeon. The surgeon is often called upon to correct motility disorders of the digestive tract, and consequently a thorough knowledge of the digestive system would provide the pediatric surgeon with essential insight. In this paper we deal with the lower digestive tract only.

Infantile Hypertrophic Pyloric Stenosis

Infantile hypertrophic pyloric stenosis (IHPS) is a motility disorder of the outlet of the stomach. It is the most common disease requiring abdominal surgery in early infancy. It was described in detail for the first time in 1888 by Hirschsprung as an entity of unknown origin. It leads to a permanent contraction of the pylorus. Ultrasound examination carried out by expert pediatric radiologists has been proven to provide a reliable diagnosis (Ball et al. 1983). Early pyloromyotomy, as first described by Ramstedt in 1912, provides a safe and simple surgical correction.

Tam (1986) has reviewed the literature extensively. IHPS has a high familial incidence, leading to genetic factors which are important for the etiology of this disease, although it is probably not congenital as it develops after birth. Neuronal immaturity and degeneration have been suggested as causative factors, but this has been refuted by other investigators. In his study of IHPS, Tam found a paucity of substance P and he regards this finding as supporting the hypothesis that substance P-containing nerves play an etiological role in IHPS. The muscle overgrowth in IHPS appeared to be a result of pure hypertrophy with no hyperplasia of muscle cells. Acetylcholinesterase staining did not reveal any gross abnormalities of the myenteric ganglia in IHPS, while neuron-specific enolase immunostaining revealed the presence of mature, well-differentiated ganglia. IHPS remains an enigma, although its surgical treatment is simple and safe, which cannot be said for all other motility disorders of the infantile gut.

Small-Bowel Dysmotility

Intestinal dysmotility after surgical repair for intestinal atresia is the result of inadequate resection of the proximal dilated segment. Nixon's work (1955) in this field demonstrated that the dilated segment is unable to contract sufficiently for the intestinal contents to move into the normally contracting distal part of the small bowel, and as such must be resected.

Intestinal dysmotility after surgical correction for gastroschisis is not uncommon. Haller and co-workers (1974) believed that the disordered peristalsis in these cases resulted from potentially reversible damage to myenteric ganglion cells. Our study of experimental gastroschisis in the chicken embryo did not reveal any such disturbance in the development or structure of the innervation of the bowel. We did find that exposure to the urine-containing allantoic fluid is a prerequisite for the development of the typical fibrous coating of the bowel wall in the chicken gastroschisis model (Klück et al. 1983). Its occurrence was directly related to an increase in the concentration of creatinine, urea, and uric acid in the allantoic fluid from the 14th day of development.

We also studied human embryos with gastroschisis, and we analyzed human amniotic fluid. The findings were in agreement with our experimental studies, revealing that the defect in the bowel wall occurs early in fetal life, while the typical fibrous coating of the bowel develops only at a later phase, after the secretion of urine into the amniotic fluid has come into effect. Finally, we investigated bowel specimens from four patients with gastroschisis. These specimens were obtained either at operation for concomitant intestinal atresia or at autospy. All four patients had suffered from prolonged intestinal dysmotility. We found severe ischemic changes of the bowel resulting in muscular necrosis. This ischemia may well be due to the small opening in the abdominal wall through which the bowel protrudes in gastroschisis, causing congestion as the bowel grows in size.

In conclusion, dysmotility of the small bowel in gastroschisis is related to fibrous coating and strangulation leading to edema and ischemia of the bowel wall. Changes in the enteric nervous system are due to transmural ischemia of the bowel and are not related to primary differentiation disturbances in the enteric ganglion cells (Tibboel et al. 1986).

Pseudo-Obstruction

A motility disorder presenting as an adynamic bowel (Duhamel et al. 1980) in premature infants may be understood as immaturity of the enteric ganglia. This condition is common in prematurity and should be handled with extreme caution. The following case provides a good illustration:

Some years ago, a male neonate with a gestational age of 31 weeks and a birth weight of 990 g, was admitted to our hospital. His abdomen was slightly distended while bowel loops and peristaltic movements could easily be discerned through his thin abdominal wall. Feeding proved difficult due to vomiting and progressive abdominal distension. Only small enemas with either oil or meglumine diatrizoate (Gastrografin) resulted in the evacuation of some meconium. Radiology revealed no abnormalities in his colon. Fourteen days after birth he was still obstructed. Then we made the mistake of taking a suction biopsy from his rectal wall. The biopsy did not reveal any anomaly of the bowel wall. However, an X-ray taken a few days later showed free air in the abdominal cavity and corrective laparotomy confirmed the diagnosis of perforation of the rectal wall just above the peritoneal fold in the pelvic cavity. The postoperative follow-up was uneventful.

This type of small-bowel dysmotility in prematurity has now become rather familiar and the therapeutic approach has become very conservative (Vinograd et al. 1983). The phenomenon "immature enteric neuron" has, however, mainly been defined on a morphologic basis using routine histological and enzyme-histochemical methods (Munakata et al. 1978). Evaluation of these patients using monoclonal antibodies raised against different differentiation markers specific for enteric neurons is needed in the future (Tibboel et al. 1987). Clinical experience shows that the motility disorder in these very premature babies is only temporary, and this suggests a maturation problem.

Colonic Dysmotility

In 1948, Swenson and Bill described their experience with a transverse colostomy for severe congenital chronic constipation. They had noted the remarkable phenomenon that patients were relieved of their symptoms only as long as the colostomy was maintained. Pressure studies led Swenson to the conclusion that these patients had a segment of colon which was without any peristaltic activity, and which had to be removed. This was first done experimentally in dogs. When such a low rectocolic resection proved feasible without producing incontinence, this operation was performed on children with most gratifying results.

The pressure studies of Swenson have been perfected, and electromanometry (Holschneider 1983) has revealed additional phenomena, such as mass contractions in the anorectal and rectosigmoidal region, as well as failure of the internal anal sphincter to respond with reflex relaxation to distension of the rectum with a balloon.

Various surgical techniques have been developed for the treatment of Hirschsprung's disease. As early as 1953, Rehbein discontinued Swenson's procedure, developing a technique whereby he could carry out a very deep resection with anastomosis via the abdomen. Duhamel subsequently developed another technique in 1960, followed by Soave in 1964 with yet another procedure. Thousands of children have undergone surgery following one or the other of these procedures. Oddly enough, the results are practically identical for all methods. Holschneider (1983) carried out an extensive literature study involving over 5000 patients to which he added his own data concerning more than 400 patients. He found that obstipation poses a constant problem in 9%–10% of these patients, while the same percentage of patients remains at risk for enterocolitis. Rehbein (1976) blames the sphincter mechanism for the postoperative complications, which according to him disappear only after a permanent reduction in sphincter pressure.

Histological investigation of the rectal wall – not manometry – became the decisive tool in the diagnosis of Hirschsprung's disease. This was initially based on a negative finding, namely, the absence of ganglion cells. This investigation requires a full-thickness rectal wall biopsy, which must be taken under complete anesthesia. When it appeared that the distal aganglionic intestinal segment contained numerous neural fibers that would stain beautifully with the aid of histochemical techniques, acetylcholinesterase staining became popular. Thanks to the work of Meier-Ruge et al. (1972), and Campbell and Noblett (1969), it became fashionable to diagnose Hirschsprung's disease on the basis of mucosal suction biopsy specimens and to regard acetylcholinesterase staining as a reliable staining technique. However, in 1981 Garrett and Howard reported that without a full-thickness biopsy they would have missed 12 cases of hypoganglionosis out of a series of 35 chronically constipated patients. They also found that the distal portion of the ganglionic part of the bowel specimen resected in patients with Hirschsprung's disease may reveal a staining pattern of hypoganglionosis identical to that found in patients with hypoganglionosis without aganglionosis. In other words, as disabling constipation cannot be related solely to aganglionosis, the need for full-thickness biopsies remains.

A formaldehyde-induced fluorescence technique has been developed to show the presence of fluorescent adrenergic nerves. This method is not commonly used, while both results and interpretation of results vary. The acetylcholinesterase-stained and fluorescent nerve fibers are commonly regarded as desperately looking for synapses in the abnormal aganglionic part of the bowel. However, no conclusive proof has yet been furnished for this premise.

Apart from cholinergic and adrenergic nerve tissue, other neurotransmitter-producing tissue has been identified in the bowel wall. This nerve tissue produces noncholinergic, nonadrenergic neurotransmitters with divergent chemical composition and function. Tam (1986) detected substance P as early as the 9th week of gestation in all levels of the fetal gut. In Hirschsprung's disease, the aganglionic colon revealed concentrations of substance P in only 15% of those with normal colon. Immunohistochemical investigation of substance P supported these findings. Other investigators reported similar findings for other neurotransmitters in Hirschsprung's disease.

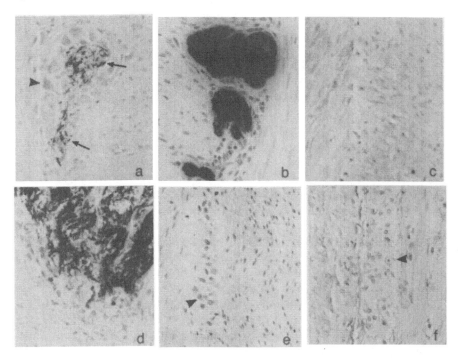

Fig. 1. a Normal bowel. *Arrowhead* indicates ganglion cell; *arrows* show normal staining of normal nervous tissue. **b** Hirschsprung's disease. Heavily stained axon bundles and absence of ganglion cells. **c** Long-segmental aganglionosis. Total lack of nervous tissue. **d** Hyperganglionosis. Heavily stained hyperplastic axon bundles. *Arrowhead* indicates surplus of ganglion cells. **e** Hypoganglionosis. Hypoplastic nervous tissue. *Arrowhead* indicates dispersed groups of small ganglion cells. **f** Pseudo-obstructed bowel. Unstained, normal nervous tissue. *Arrowhead* indicates normal ganglion cell

It is also believed that neurons can produce diverse neurotransmitters under divergent conditions. In 1981, Gershon and Erde estimated that the function of approximately 65% of the neurons in the myenteric plexus, and approximately 20% of the neurons in the submucous plexus, had not yet been identified. No major advances have been made since then.

The expertise of the pathologists is invaluable for a better understanding of Hirschsprung's disease and other related disorders of bowel evacuation. Our experimental studies, using monoclonal antibodies, may have made some contribution in this respect (Klück et al. 1984).

Two monoclonal antibodies (3G6 and NF2F11) have been raised against neurofilament isolated from normal adult brain tissue. Like all other eukaryotic cells, the nerve cell has a cytoskeleton. The diameter of the long thin axon of a neuron may be only a millionth of its length. It is obvious that without a tough intracellular support from the cytoskeleton, this axon would run a serious risk of breaking. The cytoskeleton of nerve cells consist of microtubules, neurofilaments and actin filaments. Neurofilaments consist of three different filaments of polypeptides, the so-called neurofilament triplet proteins, with respective molecular weights of 70000, 160000, and 210000.

These antibodies were used for immunohistochemical staining of tissue sections of full-thickness biopsies fixed in formalin and embedded in paraffin. We found that in paraffin sections of normal colon, both antineurofilament antibodies stained only some axons in the axon bundles of the myenteric plexus. Even less staining emerged in the submucous plexus. The ganglion cells did not stain at all (see Fig. 1a). In the sections of aganglionic colon of patients with Hirschsprung's disease, axon bundles stained heavily in the myenteric plexus. A similar staining was found in the submucous plexus (see Fig. 1b).

For a better understanding of this phenomenon, we wanted to determine on which type of nerves the antigen was located. To this effect, we used the monoclonal antibody NF2F11, studying paraffin sections of various tissues. These consisted of various spinal cord segments, spinal ganglia, cranial nerves (III–XII), striated muscle, skin, bladder, urethra, and uterus, taken from various patients (resection or postmortem material). In spinal cord, ventral and dorsal roots, spinal ganglia, and cranial nerves, all axons stained without exception. In the striated muscle sections, staining was limited to the axon bundles situated in the interfascicular connective tissue. The terminal arborization of the axon in the muscle did not stain. In the dermal biopsies, staining was limited to the subcutaneous axon bundles, and likewise to axon bundles in the adventitia of bladder, urethra, and uterus. In these three organs we also noted staining of some axon bundles in the muscular wall and even a single axon bundle in the submucosa.

Our findings support the hypothesis that the axons stained with this antibody originate outside the bowel wall, and as such are not part of the intrinsic innervation of the bowel. The heavily stained axon bundles in the myenteric and submucous plexus in the aganglionic colon in Hirschsprung's disease are extrinsic in origin. Tam (1986) believes that the proliferation of extrinsic nerves in the aganglionic colon is metabolically active, and that this plays a role in the inability of this part of the bowel to relax.

With immunohistochemical staining techniques, using monoclonal antineurofilament antibodies in combination with hematoxylin counterstaining, we have established six divergent staining patterns enabling the diagnosis of congenital neurogenic abnormalities of the bowel. These patterns (see Fig. 1) apply to: (a) normal bowel, (b) Hirschsprung's disease, (c) long-segment aganglionosis, (d) hyperganglionosis, (e) hypoganglionosis, and (f) pseudo-obstructed bowel.

Garrett and Howard (1981) reported that the distal portion of the ganglionic segment of the bowel resected in patients with Hirschsprung's disease may reveal a picture of hypoganglionosis. This prompted us to reevaluate our patients with Hirschsprung's disease, using the monoclonal antineurofilament antibody staining technique. We used the antineurofilament antibody to reinvestigate 22 patients out of a total of 108 neonates treated for aganglionosis at the Sophia Children's Hospital between 1975 and 1983. These 22 patients had suffered from disturbed defecation postoperatively. Out of the remainder that did not suffer from postoperative constipation, 17 were selected at random to serve as controls. In the problem group there were 16 cases of classical Hirschsprung's disease, four of long-segment aganglionosis, one of aganglionosis up to the cecum, and one of total colonic aganglionosis. The control group comprised 14 cases of classical Hirschsprung's disease, one of long-segment aganglionosis, one of total colonic aganglionosis, and one patient with an ultrashort aganglionic segment.

Using the monoclonal antineurofilament antibody NF2F11, we investigated available material from all 39 patients. This material consisted of ganglionic as well as aganglionic bowel specimens taken at operation (resection). The original diagnosis was confirmed in all cases. Proximal ganglionic bowel of all 17 controls appeared normal, there was normal (partial) staining of normal nervous tissue (Fig. 1a). In contrast, the ganglionic bowel of the patients with postoperative obstipation revealed the picture for normal bowel in only 4 out of 22. In 18 cases the antibody revealed the picture established for pseudo-obstruction, normal nervous tissue remained unstained (Fig. 1f). Early recognition of an abnormal staining pattern in proximal ganglionated bowel might provide early warning of postoperative complications.

In another study (Klück et al. 1987) we found that rectal biopsies of chronically constipated patients, adults as well as children, revealed the abnormal staining pattern defined as pseudo-obstruction.

These findings have led to our belief that Hirschsprung's disease, when used to denote aganglionosis of a segment of the distal colon and rectum, amounts to only part of an innervation disorder better described as neuronal dysplasia, comprising distal aganglionosis, long-segment and total aganglionosis, zonal aganglionosis, hypoganglionosis, hyperganglionosis, and pseudo-obstruction. Although the monoclonal antineurofilament antibody staining technique enables a simple and clear histochemical classification of the various types of innervation disorders of the bowel, it does not provide much insight into the enigma of etiology and pathogenesis.

Basic Aspects of Enteric Nervous System Development in Relation to Hirschsprung's Disease

An important phenomenon in embryology is cell migration. Cell migration is a central feature in the development of the nervous system. Most types of cells have a strong affinity for cells of their own kind. This affinity usually restrains cells from wandering from their site of origin. There are, however, cells that not only wander, but even undertake long migrations from their site of origin to colonize distant parts. That is precisely what neural crest cells do (Alberts et al. 1983). Neural crest cell migration has been studied in quail-chicken chimeras by LeDouarin (1982). She grafted part of the quail neural tube, including the neural crest, into a host chicken embryo. The quail cells were identified on the basis of a divergence in DNA staining as far as the structure was concerned. While quail cells have a spotted chromatin structure, chicken cells have a more diffuse structure in the nuclei. Using quail-chicken chimeras LeDouarin was able to construct a fate map of various levels of the neural crest. Cells migrate to the skin and differentiate into melanocytes; truncal neural crest cells migrate to the region of the vertebral column and the retroperitoneum to become sensory dorsal root ganglia, the ganglia of the sympathetic chain and the adrenal medulla. Vagal neural crest cells migrate to the bowel and differentiate into parasympathetic enteric neurons. Sacral neural crest cells also migrate to the bowel and give rise to enteric neurons up to the umbilicus.

To determine whether enteric neurons derive from the vagal and the sacral neural crest or from the vagal neural crest alone, we designed an experiment that interrupted the craniocaudal migration of vagal crest cells and allowed for a putative caudocranial migration of sacral neural crest cells. We transected the bowel in E4 to E7 embryos at the postumbilical level. At the time of fixation (E12) we did not observe enteric neurons in the hindgut of embryos that had undergone bowel transection at E4. In these bowels, we observed empty myenteric ganglia that contained axon bundles. The histological picture resembles that seen in cases of Hirschsprung's disease. Thus transection of embryonic bowel at early stages of development provides an animal model for Hirschsprung's disease. This offers opportunities for the study of basic mechanisms in formation of the enteric nervous system (Meijers et al. 1989).

The pathways of neural crest cell migration are lined by specific extracellular matrix molecules, e.g. fibronectin, laminin (Alberts et al. 1983; Duband and Thiery 1982). The differentiation of neural crest cells depends on the local microenvironment in the target organ.

Investigating the origin of enteric ganglia in human embryos, Okamoto and Ueda (1967) observed a craniocaudal sequence of silver-stained neuroblasts along the developing bowel. They supposed that the craniocaudal sequence reflected craniocaudal migration of neural crest cells. They speculated that the distal aganglionosis in Hirschsprung's disease resulted from an imbalance between neural crest cell migration and longitudinal growth of the bowel. We investigated this hypothesis experimentally in chicken embryos (Meijers et al. 1987a). We studied this problem by transplanting developing bowel and nervous tissue onto the chorioallantoic membrane of the chick embryo. The chorioallantoic membrane as such does not contain any nervous tissue. We obtained aneuronal (neurofilament-negative) embryonal chicken gut up to 25 days of development by culturing explants of embryonic E4 bowel. The presence or the absence of neural crest cells was determined with the HNK-1 antibody. Enteric neurons were demonstrated with antineurofilament antibodies. Neural crest cell colonization of the bowel was observed, even in advanced stages of differentiation if cocultured with the neural anlage (neural tube and neural crest). Consequently, slow migration of neural crest cells in the course of normal bowel differentiation does not necessarily lead to aganglionosis.

Recently the ischemic pathogenetic mechanism for Hirschsprung's disease was raised again (Earlam 1985). The presence of fibromuscular dysplasia of the arteries in the aganglionic colon of patients with Hirschsprung's disease supports this theory. If ischemia plays a part in the pathogenesis of congenital aganglionosis, then the ischemic insult must occur before birth. To test this hypothesis we evaluated the enteric nervous system in case of proven antenatal intestinal ischemia (intestinal atresia and meconium peritonitis) in a combined experimental and clinical study.

Enteric neurons were only absent if severe ischemic changes had occurred in all layers of the bowel in resection specimen of patients with intestinal atresia. No differences were found between small bowel and colonic atresia. Permanent or temporary local intestinal ischemia induced in chicken embryos at E16 led to atresia and stenosis of the small bowel in a considerable number of cases. Irrespective of the type of ischemia induced in these embryos, enteric neurons were only absent or pyknotic if severe ischemic changes had occurred in the bowel wall (manuscript submitted for publication). In conclusion: local intestinal ischemia during development does not lead to selective disappearance of enteric neurons.

It is known that cells of the neural crest divide and express differentiation characteristics at the same time (e.g., acetylcholinesterase activity and neurofilament proteins) (Payette et al. 1984). It is not known whether the dividing capacity of neural crest cells is restricted to the neural crest area. To study the dividing properties of neural crest cells in the developing gut, ^{3}H-thymidine was applied onto the chorioallantoic membrane. By this method all cells passing through the S-phase will incorporate the isotopes. By means of a double labeling technique of neural crest cells with HNK-1 antibodies and autoradiography, we found that migrating enteric neural crest cells still proliferate. Some cells even go through cell division after plexus formation (Meijers et al. 1987b).

Another means of studying the pathogenesis and etiology of congenital malformations of the enteric nervous system involves the use of spontaneous animal models. Lane (1966) reported megacolon in two mutant mouse strains, the piebald-lethal and the lethal-spotting strain. Both strains have an autosomal recessive gene which reduces pigmentation of the fur as well as the number of enteric neurons in the distal colon (Webster 1973, 1974). The lethal-spotted homozygotes survive longer, and it is possible to obtain litters of pure homozygotes which all develop megacolon.

To determine the timing of neural crest cell colonization of murine bowel, we cultured explants of murine embryonic bowel (of lethal-spotted and control C57B1 mice) in the renal subcapsular space. After the culture period, enteric neurons were visualized by means of acetylcholinesterase histochemistry and neurofilament immunocytochemistry. Cultured whole bowel explanted at embryonic day 9 (E9) contained enteric neurons, indicating that neural crest cell colonization of the bowel begins on or before E9. Acetylcholinesterase- and neurofilament-positive enteric neurons were consistently absent in the distal 1–2 mm of hindgut explanted at E10 to E12, indicating that neural crest cells do not colonize the entire bowel at E9. We found that neural crest cell colonization of the distal hindgut is completed at E14 (manuscript submitted for publication). A study of the development of the enteric nervous system of lethal-spotted mice using the same culture system is still in progress.

We surmise that neural crest cell colonization of embryonic murine bowel occurs in three distinctive phases: (1) migrating neural crest cells colonize the embryonic foregut and the larger part of the midgut from E7.5 to E9; (2) longitudinal growth of the bowel and neural crest cell proliferation increase the length of the innervated bowel segments from E10 to E12; (3) neural crest cells colonize the distal 1–2 mm of hindgut by active migration from E13 to E14. Disturbances during these phases may lead to diverse congenital malformations of the enteric nervous system.

Acknowledgements. Ko Hagoort, translator/stylistic editor, is thanked for assistance in preparing this manuscript. Mrs. C. C. M. van Haperen-Heuts is thanked for excellent technical assistance.

References

Alberts B, Bray D, Lewis J, Raff M, Roberts K, Watson JD (1983) Molecular biology of the cell. Garland, New York

Ball TI, Atkinson GO, Gay BB (1983) Ultrasound diagnosis of hypertrophic pyloric stenosis: realtime application and the demonstration of a new sonographic sign. Radiology 147:499–502

Campbell PE, Noblett HR (1969) Experience with rectal suction biopsy in the diagnosis of Hirschsprung's disease. J Pediatr Surg 4:410–415

Duband JL, Thiery JP (1982) Distribution of fibronectin in the early phase of avian cephalic neural crest migration. Dev Biol 93:308–323

Duhamel JF, Ricour C, Dupont C, et al (1980) L'adynamie intestinale chronique primitive a relevation neonatale. A propos de 3 observations. Arch Fr Pediatr 37:293–297

Earlam R (1985) A vascular cause for Hirschsprung's disease? Gastroenterology 88:1274–1276

Garrett JR, Howard ER (1981) Myenteric plexus of the hindgut: development abnormalities in human and experimental studies. In: Elliott K, Lawrenson G (eds) Development of the autonomic nervous system. Pitman Medical, London, pp 326–344 (CIBA Foundation symposium 83)

Gershon MD, Erde SM (1981) The nervous system of the gut. Gastroenterology 80:1571–1594

Haller JA, Kehrer BH, Shaker IJ, Shermeta DW, Wyllie RG (1974) Studies of the pathophysiology of gastroschisis in fetal sheep. J Pediatr Surg 9:627–632

Hirschsprung M (1888) Fälle von angeborener Pylorusstenose. Jb Kinderheilkunde 27:61

Holschneider AM (1983) Elektro-manometrie des Enddarms. Diagnostik und Therapie der Inkontinenz und der chronischen Obstipation, 2nd edn. Urban & Schwarzenberg, Munich

Klück P, Tibboel D, VanderKamp AWM, Molenaar JC (1983) The effect of fetal urine on the development of the bowel in gastroschisis. J Pediatr Surg 18:47–50

Klück P, Tibboel D, Molenaar JC, et al (1984) Hirschsprung's disease studied with monoclonal antibodies on tissue sections. Lancet I:652–654

Klück P, TenKate FJW, Schouten WR, et al (1987) NF2F11 staining in the investigation of severe long-standing constipation. Gastroenterology 93:872–875

Lane PW (1966) Association of megacolon with two recessive spotting genes in the mouse. J Hered 57:29–31

LeDouarin NM (1982) The neural crest. Cambridge University Press, Cambridge, UK

Meier-Ruge W, Lutterbeck PM, Herzog B, Moerger R, Moser R, Schärli A (1972) Acetylcholinesterase activity in suction biopsies of the rectum in the diagnosis of Hirschsprung's disease. J Pediatr Surg 7:11–17

Meijers JHC, Tibboel D, VanderKamp AWM, et al (1987a) The influence of the stage of differentiation of the gut on the migration of neural cells: an experimental study of Hirschsprung's disease. Pediatr Res 21:466–470

Meijers JHC, Tibboel D, VanderKamp AWM, et al (1987b) Cell division in migratory and aggregated neural crest cells in the developing gut: an experimental approach to innervation-related motility disorders of the gut. J Pediatr Surg 22:243–245

Meijers JHC, Tibboel D, VanderKamp AWM, et al (1989) A model for aganglionosis in the chicken embryo. J Pediatr Surg 24:557–561

Munakata K, Okabe I, Morita K (1978) Histologic studies of rectocolic aganglionosis and allied diseases. J Pediatr Surg 13:67–75

Nixon HH (1955) Intestinal obstruction in the newborn. Arch Dis Child 30:13–20

Okamoto E, Ueda T (1967) Embryogenesis of intramural ganglia of the gut and its relation to Hirschsprung's disease. J Pediatr Surg 2:437–443

Payette RF, Bennet GS, Gershon MD (1984) Neurofilament expression in vagal neural crest-derived precursors of enteric neurons. Dev Biol 105:273–287

Rehbein F (1976) Kinderchirurgische Operationen. Hippokrates, Stuttgart

Soave F (1964) A new surgical technique for the treatment of Hirschsprung's disease. Surgery 56:1007–1014

Swenson O, Bill AH (1948) Resection of rectum and rectosigmoid with preservation of the sphincter for benign spastic lesions producing megacolon. Surgery 4:212–220

Tam PKH (1986) An immunochemical study with neuron-specific enolase and substance-P of human enteric innervation – the normal developmental pattern and abnormal deviations in Hirschsprung's disease and pyloric stenosis. J Pediatr Surg 21:227–232

Tibboel D, Raine P, McNee M, et al (1986) Developmental aspects of gastroschisis. J Pediatr Surg 21:865–869

Tibboel D, Meijers JHC, Klück P, et al (1987) Monoclonal antibodies for diagnosis and research in enteric nervous system pathology. Dev Neurosci 9:133–143

Vinograd I, Mogle P, Peleg O, Alphan G, Lernau OZ (1983) Meconium disease in premature infants with very low birth weight. J Pediatr Surg 103:963–966

Webster W (1973) Embryogenesis of the enteric ganglia in normal mice and in mice that develop congenital aganglionic megacolon. J Embryol Exp Morphol 30:573–585

Webster W (1974) Aganglionic megacolon in piebald-lethal mice. Arch Pathol 97:111–117

Neuronal Intestinal Dysplasia

R. Rintala, J. Rapola, and I. Louhimo

Summary

A series of 21 patients with NID is presented. A histologic and histochemical picture of NID was seen in an heterogenous group of patients. NID was associated with bowel obstruction and/or perforation in six neonates and infants. One neonate died. During follow-up the bowel histology gradually normalized in four of the five patients.

NID was found incidentally in four patients with anorectal malformations and two with Hirschsprung's disease. Three patients with Hirschsprung's disease and associated NID had chronic proctitis; one patient with an anorectal anomaly had chronic obstipation and megacolon and one proctitis. Two children with multiple endocrine neoplasia 2b syndrome and chronic obstipation had typical NID in their rectum biopsies, as did a 50-year-old woman with CIIP.

The clinical heterogenity of patients with NID suggests that NID may not be a distinct clinical entity but rather a reaction of the neuronal network of the bowel wall and could be caused either by congenital or secondary factors.

Zusammenfassung

Es wird ein Bericht über 21 Patienten mit neuronaler intestinaler Dysplasie (NID) gegeben. Das histologische und histochemische Bild der NID fand sich in einer heterogenen Gruppe von Patienten. NID trat auf mit Ileus und/oder Darmperforation bei 6 Neugeborenen und Säuglingen, wovon ein Neugeborenes verstarb. Kontrolluntersuchungen zeigten bei 4 der 5 Kinder eine graduelle Normalisierung des histologischen Befundes.

NID wurde als Zufallsbefund bei 4 Patienten mit anorektalen Fehlbildungen und bei 2 mit M. Hirschsprung erhoben; 3 Patienten mit M. Hirschsprung und begleitender NID litten unter einer chronischen Proktitis, ein Patient mit anorektaler Fehlbildung litt an einer chronischen Obstipation mit Megakolon, ein anderer hatte eine Proktitis; 2 Kinder mit MEN-2b-Syndrom („multiple endokrine Neoplasien") und chronischer Obstipation zeigten in den Rektumbiopsien das typische Bild der NID, gleichfalls eine 50jährige Frau mit chronischer idiopathischer intestinaler Pseudoobstruktion (CIIP).

Die klinische Heterogenität bei Patienten mit NID legt den Schluß nahe, daß es sich bei der NID nicht um ein eigenständiges Krankheitsbild, sondern um eine Reaktionsform des neuronalen Netzes der Darmwand handelt, die sowohl durch angeborene als auch durch sekundäre Faktoren verursacht wird.

Résumé

On traite d'un groupe de 21 patients atteints de dysplasie intestinale neuronale. Il s'agit d'un groupe de patients très hétérogène présentant l'image histologique et histochimique de cette

---

Children's Hospital, University of Helsinki, Stenbackinkatu 11, SF-00290 Helsinki, Finland

affection. Elle a été rencontrée avec un iléus ou/et une perforation intestinale chez 6 nouveaux-nés et nourrissons, entraînant le décès d'un des nouveaux-nés. Les examens de contrôle ont révélé une normalisation graduelle des données histologiques.

Une dysplasie intestinale neuronale a aussi été diagnostiquée fortuitement dans le cas de 4 patients présentant des malformations anorectales et chez 2 patients atteints de maladie de Hirschsprung. Trois patients atteints de maladie de Hirschsprung et dysplasie intestinale concomitante présentaient une proctite chronique, un patient avec malformation anorectale souffrait de constipation chronique et mégacôlon, un autre patient présentait une proctite. La biopsie du rectum de deux enfants avec syndrome MEN 2b (néoplasies multiples endocrines) et constipation chronique révéla une image typique de dysplasie intestinale neuronale, tout comme chez une femme de 50 ans avec pseudo-occlusion intestinale idiopathique chronique.

Il ressort du caractère hétérogène, du point de vue clinique, des patients atteints de dysplasie intestinale neuronale, qu'il ne s'agit pas d'une entité clinique distincte mais d'un phénomène de réaction du réseau neuronal de la paroi intestinale, provoqué par des facteurs congénitaux ou secondaires.

Neuronal intestinal dysplasia (NID) is a recently described (Meier-Ruge 1971) and yet poorly understood disorder of the neuronal structure of the bowel wall. NID may appear either isolated or in connection with other congenital bowel diseases such as Hirschsprung's disease. In 1983 Fadda et al. classified neuronal dysplasias into two clinically and histologically distinguishable groups. Type A is characterized by hypoplasia or aplasia of the sympathetic innervation of the bowel wall. There are often inflammatory changes in colonic mucosa. Symptoms begin early, even neonatally, and are severe and often associated with colitis. In type B there is dysplasia of the submucous plexus with large groups of ganglion cells. These can also be found in some cases in the lamina propria of the mucosa. Symptoms are milder than in type A. The most common feature is chronic constipation, which may be associated with megacolon. Acetylcholinesterase (AChE) activity of the mucosal lamina propria and muscularis mucosae is elevated in both forms, although not as much as in Hirschsprung's disease. Combinations of the two types of dysplasia are also possible.

The connection between NID and Hirschsprung's disease is well established (Kessler and Campbell 1985; Munakata et al. 1985; Puri et al. 1977). Reports on neuronal dysplasia in anorectal malformations have not been published so far. In this paper we describe 21 cases of NID, including seven patients with anorectal malformations.

Patients and Methods

Cases of NID have been specifically sought at the Children's Hospital, University of Helsinki, for about 2 years. During this time 21 patients with a histological and histochemical picture of NID were found. Six of the patients were female and 15 male. The patients were born between 1936 and 1986. The only adult patient was a woman with a long history of functional bowel obstructions (chronic idiopathic

Table 1. Clinical features of patients with neuronal intestinal dysplasia

	Number of patients
Symptoms related to NID	
Neonatal occlusion/perforation	4
Chronic constipation	5
Symptoms possibly related to NID	
Chronic proctitis	4
CIIP	1
No clinical symptoms related to NID	7
Total	21

NID, Neuronal intestinal dysplasia; CIIP, chronic idiopathic intestinal pseudo-obstruction

intestinal pseudo-obstruction, CIIP). She was a patient of the adult gastroenterology unit of the Central Hospital of the University of Helsinki.

All 21 patients were seen during the past 2 years; in some cases older biopsy material was also reevaluated. The specimens were obtained from either mucosal or full-thickness biopsies. These were divided into two parts. One was frozen and stained for AChE by the method of Karnovsky and Roots (1964). Routine hematoxylin and eosin stain was made using the other part. All the histological and histochemical evaluations were made by one of the authors (J.R.).

Four patients with NID without associated conditions were symptomatic neonatally; two had intestinal occlusion and two bowel perforation (Table 1). One patient succumbed in sepsis after operation for a perforated cecum. Another patient with neonatal bowel perforation had to be colectomized because of severe strictures and ulcerative colitis. The colitis in the remaining rectum has been refractory to medical therapy; the patient still has colostomy at the age of 1.5 years. Two patients with neonatal occlusion had neonatal enterostomies, which were closed at the age of 1 and 1.5 years, respectively. In both cases the histological features of NID disappeared during follow-up; bowel function became normal after closure of enterostomies.

Severe constipation during the 1st year of life was the main symptom in two patients. One was treated conservatively, the other with a sphinctermyotomy. In both of these patients the initially pathological AChE staining normalized during the follow-up period (3 and 7 years, respectively).

NID associated with Hirschsprung's disease was found in five patients. Three patients of an older age group (8–17 years) had chronic proctitis, which responded favorably to intrarectal prednisolone. Two cases of NID were found in routine biopsies from the ganglionated proximal bowel taken during an operation for Hirschsprung's disease.

The typical histological picture of NID type B was found in seven cases with anorectal malformations. Five of the cases were found in routine biopsies, which were taken during posterior sagittal anorectoplasty or colostomy closure. One patient was a 17-year-old boy with chronic proctitis in his pull-through segment and another a boy aged 10 years with constipation and megacolon. All the anorectal anomalies with neuronal dysplasia were of either high or intermediate types.

The two patients with a multiple endocrine neoplasia syndrome type 2b had chronic constipation with moderate megacolon. The rectal histology was identical with NID type B.

Discussion

The clinical manifestations in our patients were most varied (Tables 1 and 2). The symptoms and early clinical course of the neonatal and infant cases (six patients) was undoubtedly related to NID. All but one of the survivors (five patients) had NID type B. During follow-up the bowel function became normal or nearly normal in these type B cases. Similar experience has been reported by Munakata et al. (1985). In their series they could not find any improvement in bowel histology in repeated biopsies. In contrast, serial biopsies from our clinically improved patients showed gradually disappearing AChE activity. The last biopsies showed normal histology. This feature suggests that along with the clinical recovery of bowel function also the neuronal network of the bowel wall may undergo maturation in patients with isolated NID. Dysmaturation or delayed maturation of the bowel innervation may be the pathophysiologic explanation of NID in neonates and infants. The association of NID with Hirschsprung's disease has been reported several times (Kessler and Campbell 1985; Munakata et al. 1985; Puri et al. 1977). NID type B was found in three older operated patients whose main complaint was

Table 2. Classification[a] of cases of neuronal intestinal dysplasia

	Number of patients
Isolated NID	
Type B	4
Type A	1
Unclassified (type A?)	1
Hirschsprung's disease and NID (all type B)	5
Anorectal malformations and NID (all type B)	7
MEN 2b-syndrome and NID (both type B)	2
CIIP and NID (type B)	1
Total	21

NID, Neuronal intestinal dysplasia; MEN, multiple endocrine neoplasia; CIIP, chronic idiopathic intestinal pseudo-obstruction
[a] After Fadda et al. (1983)

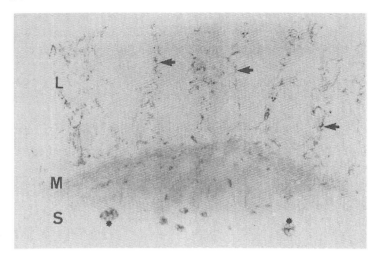

Fig. 1. Acetylcholinesterase staining of rectal mucosa of a patient with high anorectal malformation. Submucosal ganglions show high activity *(asterisks)*, and there are many esterase-positive nerve fibers in the lamina propria *(arrows)*. *L*, Lamina propria; *M*, muscularis mucosae; *S*, submucosal layer. (×120)

proctitis. Two other cases were found among the six patients who underwent operation for Hirschsprung's disease during the past 2 years. NID was observed uniformly in resected bowel proximal to the aganglionic segment. Although the number of cases is limited, these findings suggest that NID is a part of the spectrum of Hirschsprung's disease. Whether the pathophysiologic background is the same as in isolated NID, is unclear, however.

CIIP is a disease of unknown etiology. It is characterized by motor dysfunction of the intestinal tract leading to recurrent attacks of intestinal occlusions (Schuffler and Deitch 1980). Munakata et al. (1985) found NID in two children with clinically diagnosed CIIP. Our patient, a 50-year-old woman with CIIP had histological characteristics of NID type B in her resected large bowel.

Ganglioneuromatosis of the intestinal tract is a part of the multiple endocrine neoplasia syndrome type 2b (Carney et al. 1976). Some of the affected patients have megacolon. The two children with this syndrome (3 and 5 years old, respectively) had chronic constipation since infancy. Both of them had a moderate megacolon. The histology and AChE staining of the rectal biopsies were indistinguishable from NID type B.

An association of NID with anorectal malformations has not been reported before. In five of the 25 posterior sagittal anorectoplasties performed in our institute during the period 1984–1986, the full-thickness rectal biopsies which were taken during the operations revealed a histology and AChE staining pattern similar to that of NID type B (Figs. 1, 2). The finding was incidental and had no correlation to postoperative symptoms or functional results. All the patients had colos-

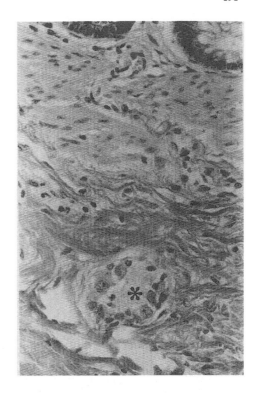

Fig. 2. An abnormally large ganglion in the submucosal layer of the same patients as in Fig. 1 *(asterisk)*. (H & E × 320)

tomas preoperatively. The colostomy (left transverse) function was normal in all three cases in which there was also NID at the colostomy site.

The series presented in this paper shows that there is a spectrum of disorders associated with NID. A strong correlation between symptoms and histology was found in the neonates and infants of our series. In these cases the disorder is without doubt congenital.

Patients in whom NID was associated with anorectal anomalies and Hirschsprung's disease can be divided into two groups. In seven cases the finding was incidental, without any apparently related symptoms. In these patients the biopsies were taken between the ages of 1 day to 4 years. In these cases the dysplasia is most probably congenital. Bioptical follow-up will show whether the neuronal dysplasia is permanent or disappears, as in the patients with isolated NID type B.

In four patients with chronic proctitis it cannot be ruled out that the NID is secondary. Reactive ganglion cell hypertrophy and hyperplasia, as well as widening and hyperplasia of the neurofilaments, have been described in colitis ulcerosa and Crohn's disease (Storsteen et al. 1953; Siemers and Dobbins 1974). Acquired NID can also not be ruled out in CIIP, where secondary changes may be caused by recurrent attacks of intestinal obstructions.

The histology and histochemistry of NID is quite uniform. However, the clinical heterogenity, which is well established in our patients, leaves many questions unanswered and warrants further studies. It is possible that NID is a common reaction of the neuronal network of the bowel wall to different factors, which may be congenital or acquired.

References

Carney JA, Go VLW, Sizemore GW, et al (1976) Alimentary tract ganglioneuromatosis – a major component of the syndrome of multiple endocrine neoplasias type 2b. N Engl J Med 295:1287–1291

Fadda B, Maier WA, Meier-Ruge W, et al (1983) Neuronale intestinale Dysplasie. Eine kritische 10-Jahres-Analyse klinischer und bioptischer Diagnose. Z Kinderchir 38:305–311

Karnovsky MS, Roots L (1964) A "direct-colouring" thiocholine method of cholinesterase. J Histochem Cytochem 12:219–221

Kessler S, Campbell JR (1985) Neuronal colonic dysplasia associated with short-segment Hirschsprung's disease. Arch Pathol Lab Med 109:532–533

Meier-Ruge W (1971) Über ein Erkrankungsbild des Kolons mit Hirschsprung-Symptomatik. Verh Dtsch Ges Pathol 55:506–509

Munakata K, Morita K, Okabe I, et al (1985) Clinical and histologic studies of neuronal intestinal dysplasia. J Pediatr Surg 20:231–235

Puri P, Lake BD, Nixon HH, et al (1977) Neuronal colonic dysplasia: an unusual association of Hirschsprung's disease. J Pediatr Surg 12:681–685

Schuffler MD, Deitch EA (1980) Chronic idiopathic intestinal pseudo-obstruction: a surgical approach. Ann Surg 192:752–761

Siemers PT, Dobbins WO (1974) The Meissner plexus in Crohn's disease of the colon. Surg Gynecol Obstet 138:39–42

Storsteen KA, Kernohan JW, Borgen JA (1953) The myenteric plexus in chronic ulcerative colitis. Surg Gynecol Obstet 97:335–339

Motility Malfunction of the Gastrointestinal Tract by Rare Diseases — Fibrosis of the Intestinal Wall

R. Daum[1], W. Nützenadel[2], H. Roth[1], and Z. Zachariou[1]

Summary

We report on two children who were admitted with chronic ileus without mechanical obstruction. In the 4-month-old female newborn, high-dose radiation was applied after extirpation of a sympathicoblastoma. Within a few years a metaplasia of the muscle coat of the small intestine developed with a resulting malabsorption syndrome. Although the damaged part of the intestine was resected, the process progressed and the child died.

In the second case, a chronic ileus developed at the age of 10 years as a result of fibrosis of the intestinal tract. Repeated laparotomies were performed, and no mechanical obstruction could be found. The most probable diagnosis is a form of scleroderma affecting mainly the alimentary tract without any skin involvment. The patient died in a severe cachexia.

Zusammenfassung

Es wird über 2 Kinder berichtet, die wegen eines Ileus ohne mechanische Obstruktion zur stationären Aufnahme kamen.

Ein Mädchen hatte im Alter von 4 Monaten eine hochdosierte Strahlentherapie nach Exstirpation eines Sympathikoblastoms erhalten. Innerhalb von einigen Jahren hatte sich eine Muskelfibrose des Dünndarms mit Malabsorptionssyndrom entwickelt. Trotz Resektion des befallenen Darmabschnitts kam es zur weiteren Verschlechterung, und das Kind verstarb.

Beim zweiten Fall entwickelte sich ein Ileus im Alter von 10 Jahren als Folge einer Darmfibrose. Wiederholt wurde laparotomiert, wobei sich jedoch keine mechanische Ursache finden ließ. Wahrscheinlich handelte es sich hier um eine Form der Sklerodermie ohne Hautbefall. Der Patient verstarb ebenfalls an den Folgen einer schweren Kachexie.

Résumé

On rapporte les cas de deux enfants hospitalisés pour iléus sans occlusion d'origine mécanique.

Une petite fille avait subi, à l'âge de 4 mois, une radiothérapie à fortes doses suite à l'excision d'un sympathicoblastome En l'espace de quelques années, elle avait développé une fibrose des muscles de l'intestin grêle et un syndrome de malabsorption. Malgré la résection du segment intestinal atteint, l'affection continua à évoluer et finit par causer le décès de l'enfant.

Dans le cas du deuxième enfant, un iléus était survenu à l'âge de 10 ans, suite à une fibrose intestinale. On procéda à plusieurs laparotomies qui ne révélèrent pas de cause mécanique. Il est probable qu'il s'agissait d'une forme de sclérodermie sans manifestation au niveau cutané. Ce patient est décédé aussi, au cours d'une cachexie majeure.

---

[1] Dept. of Pediatric Surgery and [2] Children's Hospital, University of Heidelberg, Im Neuenheimer Feld 110, D-6900 Heidelberg, FRG

The obstructive, or mechanical, ileus is generally contrasted to the paralytic ileus, which occurs as an atony either postoperatively or as a result of retroperitoneal processes. In addition to these temporary forms, chronic nonobstructive forms of ileus have also been reported. In these cases one misses the pathoanatomical substrate because the obstruction is of a purely functional nature. These forms of obstruction fall under the categories of adynamic bowel syndrome and chronical idiopathic pseudo-obstruction. Any kind of alteration in the intestinal wall can also lead to a functional obstruction. In this respect, alterations in the intestinal wall should be included in the differential diagnosis of idiopathic ileus.

We report here on two cases which fall under the category of the so-called pseudo-obstruction of the intestine.

Case Reports

Case 1

In this 4-month-old female newborn a neurogenic tumor was excised in 1969. The pathoanatomical examination showed a sympathicoblastoma with differentiated tendency to a ganglioneuroma. For unknown reasons this child was treated with radiation (total dose, 7000–8000 rad) after operation. Four years later the spine was transperitoneally set upright because of a spine deformity. Shortly after this operation the mother reported that the child could not eat well and had little appetite. The child did not thrive, and could be fed only with fluid diet.

The child underwent several examinations in different clinics, including barium meals. In 1975, 6 years and 9 months after the extirpation of the tumor, a severe malfunction in stomach evacuation was verified. In 1976, the transit time of the contrast medium was extremely slow, upon visualization of the stomach, 5.5 h after barium meal. In addition, a caliber difference in the small intestine loops was visible. The ascending colon was filled and dilated. Similar findings could be elicited in 1977. In 1980, contrast, medium could be found in the stomach even 24 h after the examination began. Narrow and wide small-intestine loops, in terms of severe dyskinesia, were seen. The duodenal, and mostly the jejunal, loops were distended and atonic. Six months after this last examination the child was first referred to our Surgical Department.

Laparotomy. At laparotomy the stomach was found extremely dilated, with a hypertrophic stomach wall. Multiple small white plaques up to 50 cm from the duodenojejunal junction were identified as cicatrices. The further intestine was smooth, and the distal ileum was affected in the same manner as the proximal jejunum. A microcolon followed the dilated ascending colon.

Treatment. Under these circumstances a gastroenterostomy and a Roux-en-Y anastomosis was performed. An atrophy of the mesenterium was present, and small cicatrices were scattered on it. Identification of the mesenteric vessel arcades was very difficult. Three weeks later the child was relaparotomized. The

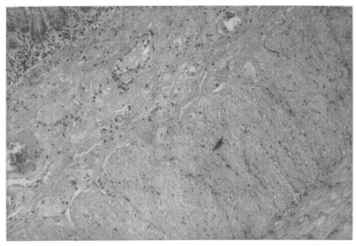

Fig. 1. Atrophic mucosa of the small bowel with fibrosis and hyalinosis of the vessel wall

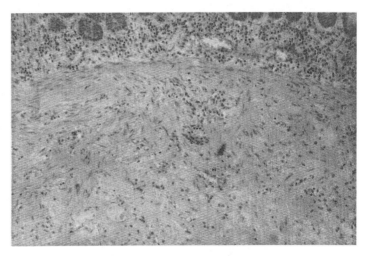

Fig. 2. Accumulation of fibrous tissue in the submucosa

previously made enteroanastomosis was contracted and occluded. An anterocolic gastoenterostoma with Braun's anastomosis was constructed after resection of the upper jejunum. The intestinal wall was edematously swollen. Within the next 3 weeks a relaparotomy was indicated because of an ileus. The adhesions were solved, and an enteroanastomosis in addition to the one present under the Braun's anastomosis was performed. A Noble's plication was also necessary.

Pathoanatomical Findings. Figure 1 shows the atrophic surface of the mucosa. The submucosa shows a severe fibrosis and hyalinosis of the vessel wall. Figure 2

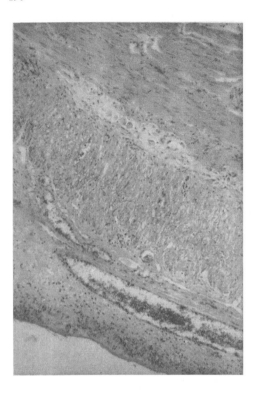

Fig. 3. Submucosal region of the small bowel with the myenteric plexus and ectatic vessels with inflammatory infiltrations

shows the accumulation of fibrous tissue in the submucosa bordering the mucosa. The submucosa is interspersed with muscular tissue. Figure 3 shows the deeper parts of the intestinal wall with the myenteric plexus in the submucosal region ectatic vessels with fibrotic and inflammatory infiltrations clearly visible.

After the operations the general condition of the child was poor, and nutrition had to be maintained by parenteral alimentation. This was achieved by construction of an arteriovenous fistula in the left forearm. Six months later the child's condition worsened, and it died in a severe state of cachexia. A postmortem examination was refused by the relatives.

Case 2

After a 10-year, uneventful early childhood this child suffered from several attacks of abdominal pain and vomiting at night. In some cases hematin was diagnosed, followed by diarrhea. In August 1973 clinical and radiological examinations were inconspicuous. In March 1974, at the age of 13, the child was laparotomized in another clinic because of suspected ileus. The distal ileum was found to be distended, and a resection of the distal ileum and cecum was performed. A mechanical obstruction was not present. The histological findings indicated no

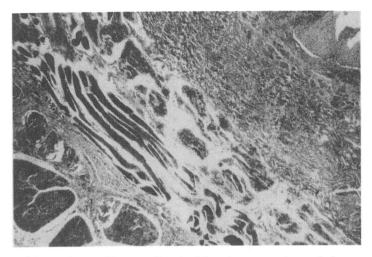

Fig. 4. Intact mucosa of the esophagus with severe fibrosis of the submucosa and muscularis

organic obstruction, but by a normal mucosa a severe thickening of the serosa. The most prominent findings were inflammation of the submucosa with lymphatic infiltration and enlargement of the mesenteric lymph nodes.

In September 1974 relaparotomy was carried out, showing intact anastomosis and no organic obstruction. The intestinal loops were found to be extremely dilated and the distal ileum thickened. A resection was not performed. In October 1974 the child was relaparotomized, and a resection of 50 cm small intestine was necessary due to adhesions. In addition, about 4 cm colon was resected due to severe hypertrophy of the wall with extremely irregular and slow peristalsis. Ten days later another operation was carried out due to ileus. A great number of adhesions were solved, and a resection of 40 cm ileum was indicated. The postoperative X ray showed fluid-air levels in the intestine with extreme motiltiy dysfunction. The transit time of barium was very slow and the contrast medium stayed in the stomach up to 11 h.

The general condition of the child became worse, even after corticosteroid therapy, cholestyramine, cholinergic drugs, metaclopramide, pancreatic enzyme substitution, and antibiotic therapy. Intermittent intravenous feeding was performed through arteriovenous fistulae in both forearms, which unfortunately obliterated within a few weeks, and on revision unusual fibrous tissue was found to have accumulated around the fistulae.

In November 1974 a relaparotomy due to adhesions was necessary. An operation after the Childs-Philipps method was performed. The therapy went on for the next 8 months, and as there was no hope of improving the condition of the child, he was discharged. The boy died in January 1976 in a severe state of malnutrition.

Postmortem Examination. The intestinal loops were adherent to each other, and the intestinal wall was paper-thin in some places. The mucosa was atrophic, and

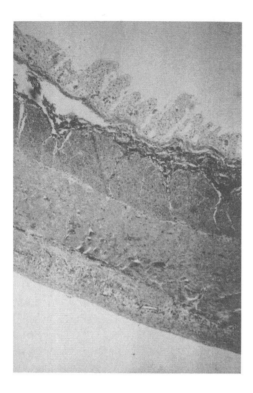

Fig. 5. Accumulation of collagen in the muscularis and serosa of the ileum

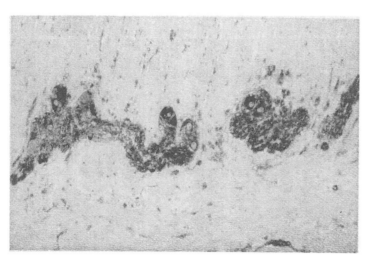

Fig. 6. Immune reaction of the neurospecific enolase in the small bowel. A granulomatosis of the myenteric plexus is present

fibrous tissue was accumulated in the submucosa and serosa. The pancreas showed a lipomatous degeneration. Slight fibrosis of the heart muscle was found, as was proliferation of the endothelium of small and very small vessels in the lungs, heart, kidney, and intestine. Figure 4 shows an intact mucosa of the esophagus but a severe fibrosis of the submucosa and the muscularis. Most prominent is the rarification and fragmentation of the intestinal wall muscle. A photomicrograph of the ileum shows thickening of the muscularis and the serosa, with accumulated collagen (Fig. 5). The mucosa is atropohic, the submucosa very thin, and the blood vessels are dilated. Figure 6 shows an interesting finding of an immune reaction of the neurospecific enolase. A ganglioneuromatosis of the myenteric plexus is present. The muscular tissue of the alimentary tract is fibrous, and in some parts ganglioneuromatosis of the submucosa is registered.

Discussion

The reason for the motility malfunction of the girl described above (case 1) is clear. Due to the high radiation that she had received, a metaplasia with replacement of the intestinal muscular coat by connective tissue occurred, especially that of the upper alimentary tract. Severe motility and coordination disorders led to chronical ileus, with a long transit time of the contrast medium, especially in the small intestine and jejunum. Although the affected parts of the intestine were resected, the process continued to the ileocecal valve. This is an extraordinary case, as we could not find anything similar to it in the literature. Today's radiation technique and radiation dosage possibly do not induce such consecutive symptoms. On the other hand, we have registered in recent years pathological changes in the form of stipples on the serosa with a tendency to adhesion. These changes cured in the form of small circatrices. The first case permits two conclusions: (a) The radiation dosage must be individually applied, the radiation field must be kept as small as possible, and the radiation of the intestine should be limited to the minimum. And (b) the radiation results in a certain degree of irreversible damage. The course is progressive and cannot be influenced by therapy. In some cases development of a carcinoma is the result of the metaplasia.

Interpretation of the second case is somewhat difficult, because the prepubertal metaplasia of the intestinal wall was established due to unknown noxa. In this case a chronic ileus without organic substrate was the major symptom.

Two groups of diseases should be included in the differential diagnosis: a clear functional disorder and a transitory malfunction which cannot be influenced. This so-called intestinal pseudo-obstructions possesses a histological substrate without known reason. These disorders may either be isolated on the gastrointestinal tract or be generalized. It is difficult, as in our case, when the symptoms are present only in the gastrointestinal tract, but generalization is not yet manifest. In other words, the gastrointestinal tract represents the first symptom of a generalized disease which pogresses to other organs in subsequent years of life.

In the second case presented here, the boy had a normal life until his 10th birthday. Then a motility malfunction of the small intestine occurred with malabsorption symptoms. Celiac syndrome was regarded an unlikely diagnosis since prolonged omission of gluten did not improve the condition. On operation, a thickening of the intestinal wall was registered. The main finding was thickening of the muscularis with replacement through connective tissue. The mucosa was atrophic, and the submucosa was fibrous with dilated blood vessels.

The immunohistological reaction with neurospecific enolase showed a proliferation of the ganglion cells of the submucosa. A functional defect of the myenteric plexus could be excluded because acetylcholinesterase activity was normal. The retractile mesenteritis was also regarded as unlikely, as there were no changes on the mesenterium (Aach et al. 1968; Black et al. 1968). The eosinophile gastroenteritis as described by Kayser (1937) could be excluded through various examinations (Klein 1970; Ureles et al. 1961). Absent were eosinophile granulomas and fleabite-like bleedings with infiltration of the intestine with eosinophile cells and eosinophilia of the liver (Kraeft et al. 1980). The histological investigation of material from our patient could not give a definite diagnosis. An idiopathic intestinal pseudo-obstruction was not identified, because in this diseases, which Naish et al. (1960) and later others (Malchanado et al. 1970; Paul et al. 1961) described, a pathoanatomical substrate does not exist.

The diagnosis of the scleroderma without or with little skin manifestation could be postulated after the postmortem examination with the multiple organ fibrosis (Heinz et al. 1963; Hoskins et al. 1962; Rodnan and Fenell 1962; Salen et al. 1966). Schuffler and Beegle (1979) described a disease with a visceral myopathy by which, in opposition to progressive, systemic sclerosis of the alimentary tract, vacuol degeneration is present. The hereditary disease can be distinguished from the progressive systemic sclerosis of the gastrointestinal tract in that a vacuolic degeneration can not be found histologically.

The boy's malnutrition could also be explained by bacterial overgrowth in the small intestine, as observed by others (Horswell et al.1961; Mc Brian and Mummery 1956; Sommerville et al. 1959). The motility disorder can lead to the establishment of an abnormal bacterial flora.

In our patients we could not find any changes on the skin, as in the case of scleroderma. We infer that the boy died before skin manifestation occurred. We can only speculate whether the disease of our patient constitutes a subcategory of scleroderma. A biopsy of the esophagus and colon should be performed for verification of possible histological changes.

References

Aach RD, Kuhn LJ, Frech RS (1968) Obstruction of the small intestine due to retractile mesenteritis. Gastroenterology 54:94–98
Black W, Nelson D, Walker W (1968) Multifocal subperitoneal sclerosis. Surgery 63:706–710
Heinz ER, Steinberg AJ, Sackner MA (1963) Roentgenographic and pathologic aspects of intestinal scleroderma. Ann Intern Med 59:822–826

Horswell RR, Hargrove MD, Peete WP, Ruffin MS (1961) Scleroderma presenting as the malabsorption syndrome. A case report. Gastroenterology 40:580–581

Hoskins LC, Norris HT, Gottlieb LS, Zamckeck N (1962) Functional and morphologic alterations of gastrointestinal tract in progressive systemic sclerosis. Am J Med 33:459–470

Kayser R (1937) Zur Kenntnis der allergischen Affektionen des Verdauungskanals vom Standpunkt des Chirurgen aus. Langenbecks Arch Klin Chir 188:36

Klein NC (1970) Eosinophilic gastroenteritis. Medicine (Baltimore) 49:299

Kraeft H, Holschneider AM, Konrad EA (1980) Obstruktive eosinophile Gastroenteritis. Paediatr Prax 23:419–425

Malchanado JE, Gregg JA, Green PA, Brown AL (1970) Chronic idiopathic intestinal pseudo-obstruction. Am J Med 49:203–212

McBrian DJ, Mummery HEL (1956) Steatorrhea in progressive systemic sclerosis. Br Med J II:1653

Naish JM, Capper WM, Brown NJ (1960) Intestinal pseudo-obstruction with steatorrhoea. Gut 1:62–66

Paul CA, Tomiyasu U, Mellin-Koff SM (1961) Nearly fatal pseudo-obstruction of the small intestine. A case report of its relief by subtotal resection of the small bowel. Gastroenterology 40:698

Rodnan GP, Fenell RH (1962) Progressive systemic sclerosis sine scleroderma. JAMA 180:97–102

Salen G, Goldstein F, Wirts CW (1966) Malabsorption in intestinal scleroderma. Relation to bacterial flora and treatment with antibiotics. Ann Intern Med 64:834–841

Schuffler MD, Beegle RG (1979) Progressive systemic sclerosis of the gastrointestinal tract and hereditary hollow visceral myopathy: two distinguishable disorders of intestinal smooth muscle. Gastroenterology 77:664–671

Sommerville RL, Bargen JA, Pugh DG (1959) Scleroderma of the small intestine. Postgrad Med 26:356–364

Ureles AL, Alschibaja T, Lodico D, Stabius SJ (1961) Idiopathic eosinophilic infiltration of the gastrointestinal tract, diffuse and circumscribed. Am J Med 30:899

Transient Functional Obstruction of the Colon in Neonates: Examination of Its Development by Manometry and Biopsies*

G. Lassmann[1], A. Kees[2], K. Körner[2], and P. Wurnig[2]

Summary

Between 1975 and 1983, 17 neonates with transient functional obstruction of the colon were studied in our surgical department. Five could be successfully treated conservatively with enemas. In the remaining 12 cases colostomy was necessary. In three cases colostomy was performed too late and the patients died. In the other nine cases rectal biopsies and anorectal manometries were performed repeatedly. In spite of clear radiological signs of colonic obstruction such as in Hirschsprung's disease in each case, and identical clinical signs, true aganglionosis could be excluded. Rectoanal manometry 4 months after colostomy showed that the situation had normalized in five cases, but was still pathological in four cases, as in aganglionosis. Of the rectal biopsies, five showed signs of immaturity of ganglionic cells and three were normal. Rectoanal manometry 12–24 months later showed normal reaction in all cases, and of the five cases with immaturity of the ganglionic cells at 4 months one was still pathologic at 12–24 months.

In eight of 12 cases the colostomy was closed without relapse of the obstruction, even on long-term follow up. Aganglionosis of the ultrashort type was excluded. In cases of severe transient functional obstruction of the colon in neonates, in which colostomy is necessary, rectoanal manometry and rectal biopsies should be performed as early as possible. Rectoanal manometry, at least, should be done before closure of the colostomy to avoid relapse of the obstruction from closing it to early: the functional disturbance may persist for several months. The term "small left colon syndrome" should be abandoned in favor of "transient functional obstruction," as the latter describes the clinical condition far better.

Zusammenfassung

Zwischen 1975 and 1983 wurden 17 Neugeborene wegen passagerer funktioneller Kolonobstruktion an unserer Kinderchirurgischen Abteilung behandelt; 5 wurden durch Einläufe geheilt. Bei 12 Fällen war die Anlage eines Kolostomas notwendig; 3mal wurde die Kolostomie zu spät angelegt, und die Patienten verstarben. Bei den anderen 9 Fällen wurden wiederholt rektale Biopsien und Manometrien durchgeführt. Trotz radiologischer Zeichen einer Kolonobstruktion vom Typ des M. Hirschsprung in allen Fällen konnte eine echte Aganglionie ausgeschlossen werden. Bei 4 Fällen ergab die Manometrie 4 Monate nach Kolostomie noch pathologische Befunde wie bei der Aganglionie; in 5 Fällen hatten sich die Befunde normalisiert. Rektale Biopsien zeigten 5mal Zeichen einer Unreife der Ganglienzellen und 3mal normale Befunde. Die rektoanale Manometrie ergab 12–24 Monate später Normalbefunde bei allen Kindern. Von den 5 Kindern, die eine Unreife der Ganglienzellen aufwiesen, ergaben sich bei einem zu diesem Zeitpunkt noch pathologische Befunde. Bei 8 Kindern konnte die Kolostomie ohne Obstruktionsrezidiv in der

---

* Supported by a grant from the Jubilee Funds of the National Bank of Austria (project number 1850)
[1] Neurological Institute of the University of Vienna, Schwarzspanierstr. 17, A-1090 Vienna, Austria
[2] Mautner-Markhof'sches Kinderspital der Stadt Wien, Baumgasse 75, A-1030 Vienna, Austria

Verlaufsbeobachtung verschlossen werden. Ein ultrakurzes Segment fand sich in keinem Fall. Bei der schweren passageren funktionellen Kolonobstruktion des Neugeborenen („small left colon syndrome"), wo eine Kolostomie notwendig wird, soll vor Verschluß des Kolostomas eine rektoanale Manometrie und eine rektale Biopsie durchgeführt werden, um ein Rezidiv der Obstruktion zu verhindern, da diese funktionelle Störung in einzelnen Fällen mehrere Monate zur Ausheilung benötigt. Der Begriff „small-left-colon-syndrome" sollte zugunsten „transient functional obstruction" aufgegeben werden.

Résumé

Entre 1975 et 1983, nous avons traité 17 nouveaux-nés hospitalisés dans notre service de chirurgie pédiatrique pour occlusion fonctionnelle transitoire du côlon. Cinq ont été guéris par des lavements. Dans 12 cas, il a fallu pratiquer une colostomie. Dans trois cas, l'intervention a été pratiquée trop tard et les patients sont décédés. Pour les 9 cas restants, on a pratiqué à plusieurs reprises des biopsies et des manométries rectales. En dépit de signes radiologiques d'une occlusion du colon de type maladie de Hirschsprung, présents dans tous les cas, on a pu écarter une véritable aganglionie. Dans 4 cas, la manométrie effectuée 4 mois après une colostomie révéla des aspects pathologiques identiques à ceux d'une aganglionie, dans les cinq autres cas, les résultats s'étaient normalisés. Des biopsies rectales révélèrent cinq fois des signes d'immaturité des cellules ganglionnaires et trois fois une situation normale.

La manométrie recto-anale, pratiquée de 12 à 24 mois plus tard, donna des résultats normaux dans le cas de tous les enfants. Chez un des cinq enfants présentant des signes d'immaturité des cellules ganglionnaires, il y avait encore à l'époque quelques résultats pathologiques. Dans le cas de 8 enfants, la colostomie a pu être fermée sans reprise d'occlusion. En aucun cas on n'a trouvé un segment ultracourt. Dans les cas d'occlusion fonctionnelle grave transitoire du côlon chez le nouveau-né ("small left colon syndrome"), renadant nécessaire une colostomie, il faut pratiquer, avant la fermeture du colostoma, une manométrie peropératoire et une biopsie rectale pour empêcher toute récidive de l'occlusion car la guérison de ce trouble fonctionnel peut, le cas échéant, s'étaler sur plusieurs mois.

Transient functional obstruction of the colon in neonates is similar in its functional behavior and effects to Hirschsprung's disease [19], involving a malfunction of the distal section of the colon. It is better known as small left colon syndrome, and other synonyms are also used (Table 1) [1, 2, 3, 5, 8, 17, 23, 26].

Table 1. Transient functional obstruction of the colon in the newborn: terminology of various authors, with partly overlapping entities

Rack and Crouch (1957) [23]	Functional intestinal obstruction in the newborn
Sieber and Girdany (1963) [26]	Functional intestinal obstruction in the newborn
Clatworthy (1956) [8]	Meconium plug syndrome
Berdon et al. (1968) [3]	Colon inertia
Ravitch (1965) [2]	Pseudo-Hirschsprung's disease
Ehrenpreis (1965) [2]	Pseudo-Hirschsprung's disease
Davis et al. (1974) [6]	Neonatal small left colon syndrome
Le Quesne and Reilby (1975) [17]	Functional immaturity of the large bowel in the newborn

The Problem

If an obstruction is identified in the neonatal period in the lower large intestine by means of a plain X-ray, the X-ray alone does not permit differentiation with certainty between congenital megacolon and transient functional obstruction of the colon [1, 2, 3, 5, 7, 14]. Hirschsprung's disease is clinically present in 15%–81% of cases already in the neonatal period [11] and is fatal in 30% of cases with conservative treatment [12, 22, 26]. Therefore in case with known or suspected Hirschsprung's disease a colostomy should be performed [11, 12, 22, 26] to decrease the rate of early fatalities.

Because small left colon syndrome or functional obstruction of the colon cannot initially be distinguished from Hirschsprung's disease and *both* can be fatal due to enterocolitis and perforation [18, 21, 26], in severe cases it is better to relieve this colonic obstruction by colostomy too. Once a colostomy has been carried out, radiological diagnosis and differentiation of aganglionosis or similar conditions is no longer possible. If Hirschsprung's disease is then excluded by biopsy the question arises: when can it be assumed that the function of the colon is sufficiently restored to avoid a relapse of the "functional" obstruction?

Rectal manometry is then the appropriate means of examination! The colostomy can be closed only if the manometry indicates a normalization, i.e., normal movements and reflexes of the anorectum [16, 28].

Methods

For anorectal manometry we apply either a simplified method developed by one of us [13] or the method used nowadays involving direct recording of the pressure curves (Fig. 1).

Peristaltic waves are produced by a separate balloon. The registration of pressure values is performed as follows: A perfusion catheter is inserted into the rectum (tip 10 cm above the analring). The pressure in the rectum at this point is registered and marked at the corresponding place on the scheme (see Fig. 1: abscissa = distance from the anal ring in cm, ordinate = intraluminal pressure in mmHg). The tip of the measuring catheter is retracted in steps of 1 cm; the intraluminal pressure at each step is registered till the level of the sphincter ani internus is reached (Fig. 1, A). At each point (Fig. 1, 10–A) the intrarectal pressure is registered and marked. Then the sphincter-relaxation reflex of the anus is induced by expanding the small balloon already placed farther up in the rectum (Fig. 1, Top). The incoming peristalsis can be checked (double catheter or double lumen), and the now decreasing pressure at the level of the sphincter ani internus is registered (Fig. 1, R: catheter in same position as in A).

For the sake of clarity and simplification no peristalsis or masscontractions [10, 24] (Fig. 1: 1) are taken up into this scheme (Fig. 1: 2). This very simple reproduction of the obtained pressure values proved to be very useful for comparing follow-up studies with the primary condition, as shown in Fig. 2a–c.

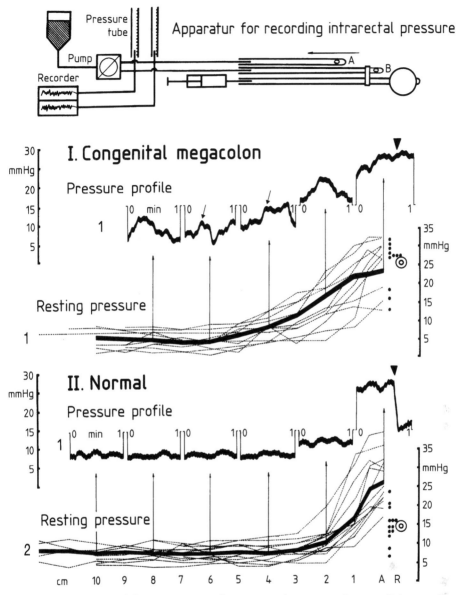

Fig. 1. Typical picture of the pressure curves from anorectal manometry in congenital megacolon *(I)* and normal cases *(II)*. The pressure curves *(1)* including registrations of the movements and mass contractions *(↗↗)* and the cleared pressure profile *(2)* are compared as described by Körner [13]. *A:* pressure in the anal ring during rest; *R:* pressure in the anal ring after sphincter-relaxation reflex is induced (▼ registration of movement). The difference in mmHg between the end of curves in A and the projected points *(R)* indicates the range of the sphincter relaxation. *Dotted lines and full points:* individual patients; *Solid lines and open circles:* mean values. *Vertical:* mmHg; *horizontal* (right to left): distance from anus *(A)* in cm. *Top:* schematic representation of the manometric device

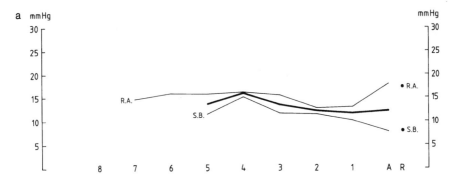
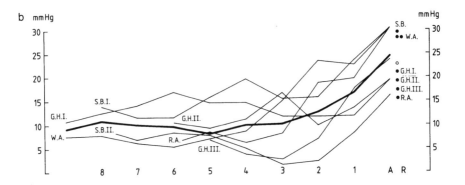
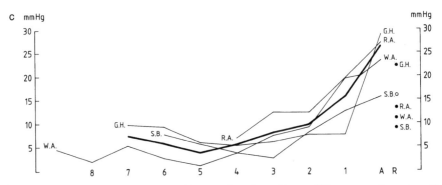

Fig. 2a–c. Pressure profiles and sphincter-relaxation reflex at different ages in patients W.A., S.B., R.A. and G.H. (Table 4). The relaxation reflex is the difference (mmHg) between the end of the curves (anus: A) and the projected points (relaxed anus: R). *Dotted lines, solid circles:* individual patients; *solid line, open circle:* mean values. *Vertical:* mmHg; *horizontal* (right to left): distance from anus (A) in cm. **a** Initial investigation. Pressure profiles as in Hirschsprung's disease: high pressure in the rectum, low tonus in the anus (A) and absent anal sphincter-relaxation reflex (R). **b** Second investigation. Maturation: lowering of pressure in the rectum, higher tonus in the anus (A) and partly absent or weak anal sphincter-relaxation reflex (R). (G.H. investigated three times, S.B. twice.) **c** Third investigation. End of maturation: normal low pressure in the rectum, high tonus in the anus (A) and well-established anal sphincter-relaxation reflex

Table 2. Group 1: conservative therapy

Patient (sex)	Vomiting	Meconium[a]	Plain X-ray	SLC	Manometry	Biopsy	Follow-up
M.F. (F)	+	2	CO	+	Profile flattened, anal reflex normal	Ø	Improved with enema
Sch.A. (F)	−	2	CO	+	Ø	Ø	Improved with enema
B.M. (M)	+	3	CO	+	Profile flattened, no anal reflex	Ø	Improved with enema
Sch.K. (F)	+	1	CO	+	Profile and anal reflex normal	Ø	Improved with enema
W.M. (M)	+	3	CO	−	Profile and anal reflex normal	Ø	Improved with enema
H.S. (M)	+	3	CO	−	Ø	Ø	Primarily improved with enemas. Relapse of CO after 16 days: emergency colostomy (perforation of cecum due to CO) 16 Sept 1975, death 17 Sept 1975
B.A. (M)	+	3	CO	−	Ø	Ø	Primarily improved with enemas. Relapse of CO: emergency colostomy (perforation of cecum) 20 Aug 1972, death 21 Aug 1972
G.J. (M)	+	2	CO	−	Profile flattened, no anal reflex	Immature ganglionic cells	Not relieved by enemas. Aspiration of gastroenteric contents and death 25 May 1977

SLC: small left colon syndrome; CO: colonic obstruction; Ø: not performed
[a] Day on which first meconium was passed

Material and Results

From the beginning of 1975 to the end of 1983 a total of 41 neonates with obstruction of the colon were observed. Twenty-four were later shown to have Hirschsprung's disease. Three of these did not have to be colostomized but could be primarily treated conservatively. The other 17 cases could be counted as neonatal functional obstruction of the colon (Tables 2–4). On X-ray all these neonates had the characteristic signs of an obstruction in the small or large intestine with delayed expulsion of meconium. They were divided into three groups.

The eight patients in group 1 (Table 2) received conservative treatment. In seven cases a meconium plug was passed by enema. The clinical development of cases with primarily conservative treatment employing one or more enemas is shown in Table 2. This was successful in five cases without further measures. In the remaining three cases, however, death resulted from persevering too long

Table 3. Group 2: colostomy with normal manometry and normal histology

Patient (sex)	Vomiting	Meconium[a]	Plain X-ray	SLC	Manometry	Biopsy	Follow-up
W. Th. (M)	+	0/2	CO	–	1. Profile and anal reflex normal 2. Profile and anal reflex normal	After 4 months, normal ganglionic cells and cholinesterase	Colostomy 4 Aug 1978, closure 17 Sept 1979
D. M. (F)	+	2	CO	–	Profile and anal reflex normal	1. Normal cholinesterase, slight hypoganglionosis and hyperplasia of fascicles 2. Enriched immigration of ganglionic cells	Colostomy 6 Jul 1979, closure 11 Mar 1980 (athyreosis treated)
M. N. (F)	+	2	CO	–	Profile flattened, anal reflex normal	Normal pattern of innervation; later possibly decreased (hypoganglionosis)	Colostomy 25 Jan 1973, closure 28 Jan 1974
W. A. (M)	+	3	CO	–	Profile and anal reflex normal	Normal pattern of innervation, normal cholinesterase	Colostomy 23 May 1977, closure 27 Sept 1978

Abbreviations as in Table 2

[a] Day on which first meconium was passed (0/2, none passed till colostomy on 2nd day)

Table 4. Group 3: colostomy with manometry and histology showing maturation

Patient (sex)	Vomiting	Meconium[a]	Plain X-ray	SLC[b]	Manometry	Biopsy	Follow-up
W.A. (M)	+	2	CO	+	1. Flattened profile, weak anal reflex (10 Feb 1975) 2. Normalized profile and anal reflex (12 Dec 1976)	Normal ganglionic cells	First colostomy 31 Aug 1975, closure 19 Sept 1975. Relapse of CO perforation: second colostomy 25 Sept 1975, second closure 25 Oct 1976
S.B. (F)	+	2	CO	+	1. No profile, no anal reflex (4 Apr 1984) 2. Flattened profile, weak anal reflex (4 Jun 1980)	Incomplete immigration of ganglionic cells	Colostomy 21 Nov 1983; after 3 weeks not yet closed
R.A. (F)	+	1	CO	+	1. No profile, no anal reflex (1 Jun 1980) 2. Flattened profile, weak anal reflex (1 Mar 1981) 3. Normalized profile and anal reflex (24 May 1982)	1. Incomplete immigration 2. Undifferentiated ganglionic cells; delayed immigration of ganglionic cells (see Fig. 4A–C)	Colostomy 7 Dec 1979, closure 2 Mar 1981
G.H. (F)	+	2	CO	+	1. Flattened profile, no anal reflex (3 Jun 1977) 2. Flattened profile, no anal reflex (4 Nov 1977) 3. Normalized profile and anal reflex (9 Mar 1978)	1. Undifferentiated ganglionic cells 2. Fully differentiated ganglionic cells (see Fig. 5A, B)	Colostomy 30 May 1976, closure 21 Feb 1978
A.A. (F)	+	2	CO	+	Anal reflex after 4 months weak, profile flattened (15 Dec 1976)	Undifferentiated ganglionic cells	Colostomy 2 Sept 1976 (age 2 months), closure 10 Jun 1977

Abbreviations as in Table 2
[a] Day on which first meconium passed
[b] Shown by barium enema

with conservative treatment. In two of these (H.J. and B.A.), perforations were found in the caecum and ascending colon. In the third case (G.J.), death followed aspiration of gastrointestinal contents during an existing obstruction of the colon. The diagnostic possibilities in these three patients were of course limited, but they exemplify the problem of the so-called "hidden mortality" and therefore cannot be omitted.

In the four cases comprising group 2 (Table 3) a colostomy was carried out. Manometry and histology (histochemical examination) showed normal conditions, so the colostomy could be closed again.

In the five cases of group 3, both manometry (Table 4, Fig. 2a, b) and histochemical analysis of the biopsies showed pathological changes. The conditions returned to normal after varying lengths of time (Table 4, Fig. 2c). The colostomy was then closed, and the children have not suffered from bowel-obstruction since. Only with one child, who moved away, could the treatment not be completed. In one case (W.A., Table 4 and Fig. 2b, c) a colostomy had to be performed a second time, after a relapse of the colonic obstruction because the first colostomy had been closed before the rectoanal function had been proved. Only after 1 year was the colonic function (i.e., the sphincter-relaxation reflex) normalized, allowing the second colostomy to be closed. Since then, however, this child has also remained free of symptoms [16, 28].

Discussion

The case histories showed clinically consistent signs, such as X-ray evidence of obstruction of the colon, rejection of nourishment, bile-stained vomiting and delayed passing of meconium. In the neonatal period it is not possible to identify Hirschsprung's disease with certainty by barium enema of the colon, because the complete picture of the megacolon with a narrow segment and a transitional zone develops only later [4, 14, 22, 27]; in most of our cases, therefore, a barium enema for the purpose of diagnosis was not administered in the early neonatal period. Initial treatment was primarily conservative, with one or more enemas. This was continued if soon successful; otherwise a colostomy was performed. Based on our clinical experience and that of others [11, 22], primary colostomy gives more favorable, results, as shown by the small number of fatalities, in which we could not identify Hirschsprung's disease but who died with the clinical picture of Hirschsprung's enterocolitis, which is well known [12, 22]. These findings are similar to those of others [18, 21, 25]. As megacolon cannot develop in Hirschsprung's disease primarily treated by colostomy, it is clear that also in these cases of "small left colon syndrome (or transient functional obstruction)" the radiological changes in the colon cannot indicate later normalization. In other words, since in cases of Hirschsprung's disease no megacolon can develop after an early colostomy, neither, in these cases, can primary dilatation of the upper parts of the colon and later normalization in the caliber of the colon (i.e., disappearance of the small left colon syndrome) be taken as evidence of normalization from the functional point of view.

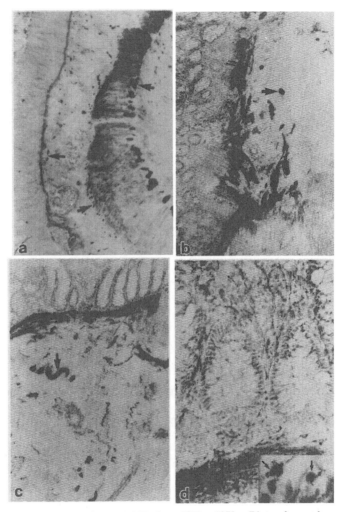

Fig. 3a–d. Two patients from group 2. **a, b** Patient M.N., born 30 Dec 1972. **a** Biopsy from colostomy 25 Jan 1973: all plexuses (Auerbach's, Meissner's and profundus; *arrows*) normal. × 60. **b** Rectal biopsy 12 Dec 1973 (L 80/73): hypoganglionosis, otherwise normal pattern of innervation. *Arrow:* ganglionic cells; *double arrow:* muscularis mucosae. × 60. **c, d** Patient D.M., born 15 May 1979. **c** Rectal biopsy on 19 Sept 1979 (L 79/79): hypoganglionosis, some larger nerve fascicles *(arrow)*, some slight hyperplasia with normal cholinesterase activity (× 120). **d** Rectal biopsy 27 Feb 1980 (L 19/80). Increased immigration by ganglionic cells in the submucosal plexus *(arrow)*, persistent discrete hyperplasia of nerve fascicles in the submucosa (× 400). **a–d** Histochemical staining of acetylcholinesterase activity, magnification as indicated

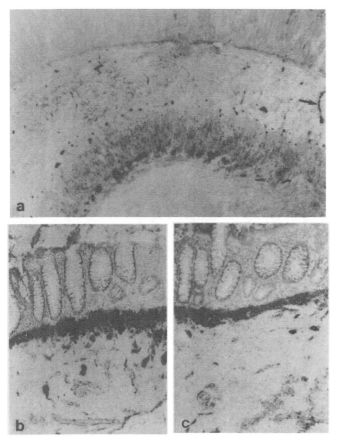

Fig. 4a–c. Patient R.A. from group 3, born 6 Dec 1979. **a** From colostomy (7 Dec 1979, first day of life), delayed immigration of ganglionic cells into the myenteric and submusosal plexus. Clear migration trace *(arrow)* from the plexus profundus to the not yet completely developed submucosal plexus × 60. **b** Rectal biopsy 7 Feb 1980 (L 11/80): ganglionic cells small, not yet fully differentiated; migration not yet complete. × 120. **c** Rectal biopsy 27 Feb 1981 (L 26/81): migration of ganglionic cells into the submucosal plexus complete, as demonstrated by lack of ganglionic cells in the deeper layers of the submucosa; probably still incomplete differentiation of the small ganglionic cells. × 120

Consequently, two steps must be taken for diagnosis: First, a biopsy of the mucous membrane from the rectum for the purpose of histochemical examination must be carried out. If this shows clear aganglionosis the case is to be treated as one of Hirschsprung's disease. If, however, it shows growth disturbance, such as decreased or undeveloped cells, or even a normal population of ganglionic cells, the case should be regarded as one of neonatal functional obstruction of the colon.

Second, *manometry* must then be used to check the peristalsis and the reflex action of the anal sphincter. Closure of the colostomy is indicated and allowed

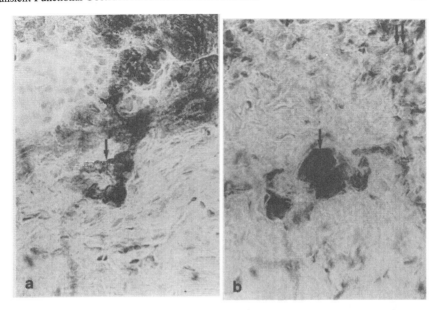

Fig. 5a, b. Patient G.H. (from group 3, born 27 May 1976. **a** Rectal biopsy 8 Jun 1977 (L 64/77): ganglion of the submucosal plexus with small, not yet differentiated ganglionic cells *(arrow)*. *Double arrow:* muscularis mucosae. **b** Rectal biopsy 2 Sept 1977 (L 90/77): ganglion of the myenteric plexus with fully differentiated ganglionic cells *(arrow)*. *Double arrow:* muscularis mucosae. Histochemical staining of acetylcholinesterase activity, × 700

only when the sphincter-relaxation reflex is normal or becomes normal again. In group 2 the manometric values and the histology were normal from the first examination (Table 3, Fig. 3a–d) and the colostomy could be closed without delay.

In contrast, in group 3 (Table 4), normalization, both manometric (Fig. 2a–c) and histological (Figs. 4, 5) came at a later time. After this period the colostomy could be closed safely without any problems. In detail, manometry offers two criteria for discrimination:

1. The pressure profile and the sphincter-relaxation reflex (Figs. 1 and 2a–c).
2. With suitable equipment, the pattern of movements in the distal region of the colon and the rectum (Fig. 1: 1). The judgement of the latter demands much more training and practice, the first allows better comparison of examinations from different times.

Figure 2b, c shows normalization of an initially poor sphincter-relaxation reflex in four patients from group 3. These patients also showed histological changes which improved (Fig. 5A, B).

Histological Problems

Hypoganglionosis

Not only do hypoganglionoses involve uncommon malformations, but comparative information about them is very difficult to obtain. A valuable neuropathological examination is possible only with the help of certain methods, mostly carried out only in centers with special experience in this kind of clinical and neurological evaluation. To illustrate the variations in the data we can compare the findings of Sieber and Girdany [26], who identified six hypoganglionoses among 70 aganglionoses from 1524 patients, and our five hypoganglionoses among 101 aganglionoses and 44 hypoganglionoses among 701 clinically preselected patients. The differences in frequency are certainly influenced by the appropriate correlation of the clinical preexamination with the neurohistological examination [9, 15]. Basically, three different forms of hypoganglionosis can be distinguished:

1. *Physiological hypoganglionosis* in the lower rectum and in the final stage of the immigration of the ganglionic cells. This is clinically significant only if the extent of the affected zone exceeds a certain size. If the state becomes irreversible, therapy is inevitably necessary.

2. *Hypoganglionosis with defective immigration* of ganglionic cells, which can also be observed in other sections of the intestine. This was the case in one of our patients from group 3 (R.A., Table 4 and Fig. 4A–C). Here it must be clarified whether or not there has been a general halt to immigration with no expectation of improvement.

3. *Regionally limited hypoganglionosis* in the rectum due to incomplete immigration at the time of birth. In this case healing of the obstruction can be expected, especially if the pattern of the nervous plexus in the colostomy (biopsy) is normal (Fig. 3a–d, cases M.N. and D.M. in Table 3).

In three of our cases the hypoganglionosis was combined with the presence of longer and larger nerve fascicles in the submucosa. These showed normal cholinesterase activity. In another case [15, 16] there was slight neural hyperplasia, limited locally to the muscularis mucosae and the lower third of the mucous membrane, with a slight increase of cholinesterase activity. It cannot be established, however, from the few cases analyzed so far, whether in such cases there is a combination of a forme fruste in a very short aganglionic segment and a hypoganglionosis. Further clinical and neuropathological surveys are necessary to ascertain to what extent in these cases a relationship exists with the ultrashort (aganglionic) segments [1, 20] often diagnosed after a longer period of illness in older children.

Disturbance of Maturation

As shown first by Emery [9] and then by our group [16], a disruption in the development of ganglionic cells is occasionally responsible for the clinical symptoms and picture of congenital megacolon. The case of our own [16] did not show any cause for such a disturbance. At present it is not possible to make a prognosis because of the small number of cases.

A delay in maturation is sometimes combined with a disturbance in immigration of ganglionic cells to the end of the intestinal tract. As in post-partum (delayed) immigration of the ganglionic cells to this region, the differentiation continues until an uncertain time after birth, at which time the functional obstruction is released. Conservative therapy with appropriate neurohistological control is thus appropriate (Fig. 5 and Table 4, patient G.H.).

Conclusions

In those cases of neonatal obstruction of the colon which cannot be influenced by conservative treatment or therapy, primary colostomy should be carried out. Exact histological and manometric analysis is necessary, first to identify the illness as Hirschsprung's disease, hypoganglionosis, disturbance in development or functional obstruction of the colon without histological changes, and second to determine by means of manometry the correct time at which to close the colostomy so as to avoid a relapse of the obstruction.

References

1. Bentley JFR (1964) Some new observations on megacolon in infancy and childhood with special reference to the management of megasigmoid and megarectum. Dis Colon Rectum 7: 462–470
2. Bentlcy JFR, Nixon HH, Ehrenpreis T, Spencer B (1966) Seminar on Pseudo-Hirschsprung's disease and related disorders. Arch Dis Child 41:143
3. Berdon WE, Slavis TL, Campbell JB, Baker DH, Haller JO (1977) Neonatal small left colon syndrome: its relationship to aganglionosis and meconium plug syndrome. Radiology 125:457
4. Bodian M, Stephens FD, Ward BCH (1949) Hirschsprung's disease and idiopathic megacolon. Lancet I:6–11
5. Davis WS, Campbell JB (1975) Neonatal small left colon syndrome. Am J Dis Child 129: 1024
6. Davis WS, Parker-Allen R, Favara BE, Slavis TL (1974) Neonatal small left colon syndrome. Am J Roentgenol Rad Ther Nucl Med 322–326
7. Ehrenpreis T (1966) Some newer aspects on Hirschsprung's disease and allied disorders. J Pediatr Surg 1:329–337
8. Ellis DG, Clatworthy HW (1966) The meconium plug revisited. J Pediatr Surg 1:54
9. Emery JL (1973) Colonic retention syndrome (megacolon) associated with immaturity of intestinal intramural plexus. Proc R Soc Med 66:222
10. Hyatt RB (1951) The pathologic physiology of congenital megacolon. Ann Surg 133:313
11. Klein MD, Coran AG, Wesley JR, Drongowski RA (1984) Hirschsprung's disease in the newborn. J Pediatr Surg 19:370
12. Kleinhaus S, Boley SJ, Sheran M, Sieber WK (1979) Hirschsprung's disease: a survey of the members of the surgical section of the American Academy of Pediatrics. J Pediatr Surg 14: 588
13. Körner K (1979) Eine vereinfachte Methode der anorectalen Manometrie. A simplified method of anorectal manometry. Z Kinderchir 28:113–120
14. Kottmeier PK, Clatworthy HW (1955) Aganglionic and functional megacolon in children, a diagnostic dilemma. Pediatrics 36:572

15. Lassmann G (1977) Light microscopic examinations of the local nervous system in the intestine. Proceedings of XVIII International Congress of Neurovegetative Research, Tokyo, 4–6 November, pp 32–47
16. Lassmann G, Wurnig P (1980) Klinische und neurohistologische Aspekte der Obstipation im Säuglings- und frühen Kindesalter. Wien Klin Wochenschr 92:420–433
17. Le Quesne GW, Reilby BJ (1975) Functional immaturity of the large bowel in the newborn infant. Radiol North Am 13:331
18. Nixon GW, London VR, Stewart DR (1975) Intestinal perforation as a complication of the neonatal small left colon syndrome. Am J Roentgenol 125:75
19. Nixon HH (1972) Problems in the diagnosis of Hirschsprung's disease. Pädiatrie Pädol [Suppl 2]:23
20. Orr JD, Scobie WG (1983) Presentation and incidence of Hirschsprung's disease. Br Med J 287:1671
21. Philippart AI, Reed JO, Georgeson KE (1975) Neonatal small left colon syndrome. J Pediatr Surg 10:733
22. Polley Th Z, Coran AG (1986) Hirschsprung's disease in the newborn, an 11-year experience. Pediatr Surg Intern 1:80–83
23. Rack FW, Crouch WL (1957) Functional intestinal obstruction in the newborn. Bull NY Acad Med 33:175
24. Schärli AF (1981) Die Verwandten des Herrn Professor Hirschsprung. Pädiatrie Pädol 16: 451–458
25. Schärli Af, Meier-Ruge W (1981) Localized and disseminated forms of neuronal dysplasia mimicking Hirschsprung's disease. J Pediatr Surg 16:164
26. Sieber WK, Girdany BR (1963) Functional intestinal obstruction in newborn infants with morphologically normal intestinal tracts. Paediatr Surg 53:357
27. Willich E (1972) Röntgendiagnostik der Hirschsprung'schen Krankheit im Neugeborenenalter und bei atypischen Fällen. Pädiatrie Pädol [Suppl 2]:7
28. Wurnig P (1986) Chronische Obstipation im Kindesalter – nur crux medici oder diagnostische Fallgrube? Wien Med Wochenschr 136:247–253

Total Colonic Aganglionosis

G. Menardi and J. Hager

Summary

A rare complication after ileorectostomy for total aganglionosis of the colon is demonstrated. Eight years after the operation fistulae between rectum and sacrum appeared. Other cases from the literature are mentioned.

Zusammenfassung

Eine seltene Komplikation nach Ileorektostomie wegen totaler Aganglionose des Kolons wird vorgestellt. Acht Jahre nach dem Eingriff traten Fisteln zwischen Rektum und Sakrum auf. Entsprechende Fälle aus der Literatur werden erwähnt.

Résumé

Les auteurs décrivent une complication rare après iléorectostomie dans un cas d'aganglionose totale du côlon. Il y a eu formation d'une fistule entre rectum et sacrum, 8 ans après l'opération. Il est fait mention des autres cas présentés dans la littérature.

Material and Methods

A total of 31 cases of Hirschsprung's disease were treated in our department, eight with total colonic aganglionosis. Of these eight patients three died. One death occurred 15 days after cecostomy; enterocolitis and perforations of the small bowel had led to peritonitis and sepsis. One extremely dystrophic child who was operated rather late at 11 months of age died intraoperatively of malignant hyperthermia; the cause of dystrophy was a fistula between jejunum and transverse colon. The third child died of gas gangrene 12 h after ileostomy.

Five children with total aganglionosis are still alive. In each of these cases, primarily a ceco- or ileostomy was performed. (We use the combined method of State and Rehbein.) The final operation was done at the age of 6 months. In one patient 30 cm of small bowel was interposed isoperistaltically between cecum and rectum. All children are under permanent supervision as outpatients. All but one

---

Department of Pediatric Surgery, University Hospital for Surgery, A-6020 Innsbruck, Austria

show normal development. Three children between the ages of 2 and 6 years had a sphinctermyectomy because of repeated spells of enteritis; nevertheless, two still suffer from intermittent enteritis. The feces of the other children are rather soft, but none is soiling or incontinent.

Late Complication

Recently we had an interesting late complication, the outcome of which is still uncertain. A 9-day-old boy underwent laparotomy because of ileus; two siblings had died elsewhere of "bowel obstruction." Biopsies showed aganglionosis up to the ileum, and an ileosotomy was performed. At the same time the colon was removed up to the splenic flexure. Six months later an ileorectostomy was carried out, followed by an uneventful recovery. Some months ago the boy, now 9 years old, developed a tender, pasty swelling over the sacral region, but this subsided after 1 week. Barium enema showed wide anastomosis and several fistulae in the sacral direction (Fig. 1). A biopsy from the anastomotic region could not exclude a terminal ileitis (Crohn's disease). Conservative therapy with salazosulfapyridine and phoscortril enemas supposedly led to the closure of the fistulae, but another barium enema 3 months later showed them again, as well as osteomyelitis of the sacrum and air in the sacral canal (Fig. 2). At this point an ileostomy was performed. Now, 6 months later, the fistulae are smaller, but still present.

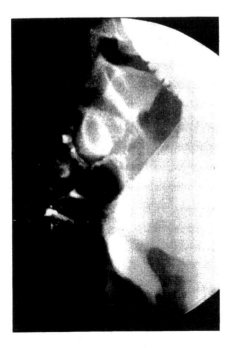

Fig. 1. Fistulae from ileorectal anastomosis toward the sacrum and into sacral canal, as shown by barium enema

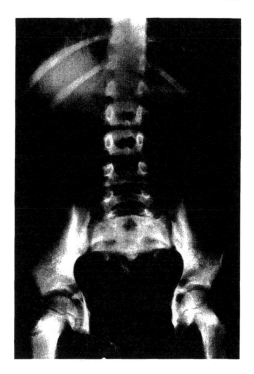

Fig. 2. Sacral osteomyelitis

Discussion

Fistulae are one of the rarest complications following operations for Hirschsprung's disease. Joppich, in a review of the literature (1982), found six authors reporting ten cases: fistulae between rectum and urethra, vagina, bowel, skin, and (like the case mentioned above the sacrum leading into the sacral canal (Table 1). According to the literature, the fistulae were usually oversown, but in the case resembling ours an ileostomy was performed. There was no information about a later closure. Noteworthy is the late appearance of the fistulae, usually after 3–5 years; in our case they appeared 8 years after operation.

Table 1. Reported fistulae after operation for Hirschsprung's disease

Author		Region
Bailie et al.	(1971)	Rectosacral
Deodhar et al.	(1973)	Rectojejunal
Jenny et al.	(1975)	Rectoileal
Baranowicz	(1977)	Rectoperineal
Puri and Nixon	(1977)	Rectovaginal
Grosfeld	(1978)	Rectourethral "fistula in ano"

References

Bailie IR, Mahour GH, Walter LE, Gwinn JL (1971) An unusual complication after Duhamel operation for Hirschsprung's disease. Int Surg 55:192–195
Baranowicz B (1975) The results of Soave's operation for Hirschsprung's disease. Z Kinderchir 20:49–56
Deodhar M, Sieber WK, Kiesewetter WB (1973) A critical look at the Soave procedure for Hirschsprung's disease. J Pediatr Surg 8:249–254
Grosfeld HL, Ballantine VN, Csiesko JF (1978) A critical evaluation of the Duhamel operation for Hirschsprung's disease. Arch Surg 113:454–460
Jenny P, Penner H, Herzog B (1975) Innere Fisteln beim operierten primär nicht diagnostizierten Morbus Hirschsprung. Helv Chir Acta 42:591–593
Joppich I (1982) Late complications of Hirschsprung's disease. In: Holschneider A (ed) Hirschsprung's disease. Hippokrates, Stuttgart, pp 258–259
Puri P, Nixon HH (1977) Long-term results of Swenson's operation for Hirschsprung's disease. Progr Pediatr Surg 10:87–96

Surgical Management of Chronic Intestinal Pseudo-obstruction in Infancy and Childhood

E. W. Fonkalsrud, H. A. Pitt, W. E. Berquist, and M. E. Ament

Summary

Chronic intestinal pseudo-obstruction is an uncommon cause of repeated obstruction in children of undetermined etiology, often leading to repeated laparotomies and early death. TPN combined with venting gastrostomy provides sufficient calories for growth and minimizes the need for operations and/or hospitalizations. Seventeen children managed with these techniques experienced a sixfold decrease in the number of hospitalizations, and more than a tenfold decrease in the number of laparotomies for obstruction compared to the period before routine use of TPN and gastrostomies. Oral feedings are encouraged whenever possible.

Zusammenfassung

Die chronische intestinale Pseudoobstruktion ist eine seltene Ursache für rezidivierende Darmobstruktionen bei Kindern mit ungeklärter Ätiologie, die häufig zu wiederholten Laparotomien und frühem Tod führt. Die totale parenterale Ernährung erlaubt in Kombination mit einer Entlüftungsgastrostomie eine ausreichende Kalorienzufuhr und reduziert die Notwendigkeit einer Operation oder Hospitalisation auf ein Minimum. Im Vergleich zu der Zeit vor der Routineanwendung der totalen parenteralen Ernährung und Entlüftungsgastrostomie konnte bei 17 Kindern, die mit diesen Methoden behandelt wurden, die Zahl der Hospitalisation um das 6fache und die Zahl der Laparotomien wegen Obstruktion um mehr als das 10fache gesenkt werden. Wenn immer möglich, sollen die Patienten zusätzlich oral ernährt werden.

Résumé

La pseudo-occlusion intestinale chronique est une cause rare d'occlusions récidivantes chez les enfants. Son étiologie n'est pas déterminée avec certitude, elle exige des laparotomies répétées et cause le plus souvent le décès précoce. Une alimentation entièrement parentérale, associée à une gastrotomie de ventilation permet d'administrer suffisamment de calories et réduit au minimum la nécessité d'une opération et d'une hospitalisation. Pour 17 enfants traités par cette technique, le nombre des hospitalisations a été inférieur de 6 fois et celui des laparotomies pour occlusion de 10 fois, par comparaison avec ce qui se serait produit à l'époque où cette alimentation entièrement parentérale associée à une gastrotomie de ventilation n'était pas pratiquée.

Chaque fois que c'est possible, il est souhaitable que ces patients soient aussi nourris par voie orale.

Departments of Surgery and Pediatrics, UCLA School of Medicine, Los Angeles, CA 90024, USA

Chronic intestinal pseudo-obstruction is a rare disorder in infancy and childhood which has been recognized with increasing frequency during the past several years. The condition is characterized by recurrent attacks of abdominal pain, distention, emesis, weight loss, and multiple hospitalizations for obstructive episodes. Changes in diet, various medications, and operations to remove or bypass segments of intestine have frequently been ineffective. As a result, most of these patients have eventually died of malnutrition. However, with the development of total parenteral nutrition (TPN) during the past 15 years, the nutritional requirements of children with pseudo-obstruction have been managed effectively. Despite this advance, however, many of the patients have continued to experience abdominal pain, distention, and emesis and have required repetitive nasogastric intubation and hospitalizations. Therefore, in an effort to maintain nutrition and to avoid severe obstructive episodes, patients with chronic intestinal pseudo-obstruction have recently been managed with both home TPN and a "venting" gastrostomy.

Patients and Methods

From 1973 through 1986, 26 patients (17 under 21 years of age) with chronic intestinal pseudo-obstruction who were treated at the UCLA Medical Center received long-term TPN. Fifteen of these 17 children were also managed with gastrostomies. At the initiation of treatment, the mean age of the 17 children was 5.6 years. Seven of the children were 2 months old or younger when TPN was started, and six were 3 months old or younger when a venting gastrostomy was placed. Ten of the 17 children were female. Prior to referral to the UCLA Medical Center, the 17 children required 44 hospital admissions for obstructive episodes. Eleven children had also undergone 37 laparotomies for what was often presumed to be mechanical obstruction. Moreover, five of the children had undergone unsuccessful trial of metoclopromide hydrochloride.

The presenting symptoms of children with intestinal pseudo-obstruction included distention in 94%, emesis in 53%, constipation in 59%, weight loss in 41%, diarrhea in 47%, abdominal pain in 30%, and dysphagia in 30%. Thus, the most frequent presenting symptoms were abdominal distention, constipation, and emesis. In addition to having a history of obstructive episodes that were repetitive or present since birth, the diagnosis of pseudo-obstruction was confirmed in all children by typical roentgenograms of the abdomen and upper gastrointestinal tract and small-bowel series. These roentgenograms in each case demonstrated one or more of the following findings: esophageal dilatation and motility disorder, delayed gastric emptying, dilated small intestine with delayed transit time, and massive colonic dilatation. A barium enema was also performed in 15 children to exclude the likelihood of Hirschsprung's disease, malrotation with midgut volvulus, internal hernias, and various other anomalies. Six children underwent upper gastrointestinal tract endoscopy. Intestinal biopsy specimens either at surgery or during endoscopy were obtained from all of the children and showed no apparent mucosal, muscular, or nerve disorder on standard light microscopy. Esophageal manometry was performed on ten children. Radionuclide gastric emptying studies were performed on four children.

On the basis of these studies, motility problems were apparent in the esophagus in 76% of the children, in the stomach in 59%, in the jejunum and ileum in 76%, and in the colon in 41%. The distribution of motility problems was variable, the most frequent pattern involving the esophagus, stomach, and small intestine which occurred in six children. None of the children evaluated in this study had isolated colonic pseudo-obstruction. Symptoms from reflux esophagitis were those of the most frequent associated illness. This problem was diagnosed in five children. Five children had associated neurogenic bladders, six having one or more urinary tract infections.

All 17 children received TPN at home for a mean of 62.4 months (range, 4–102 months). Parenteral nutrition solutions provided calories with hypertonic glucose, protein, and fat emulsions. During the 12 years of treatment, the protein source has changed, with casein hydrolosates being used in earlier years and amino acid solutions being employed more recently. Once fat emulsions became available, all children received intravenous fat twice a week. Trace metals and vitamins were also included in standard solutions, and electrolytes were added according to the needs of the individual patients. Fifteen of the 17 children also underwent tube gastrostomies. The procedure was performed by means of laparotomy using the standard STAMM technique. In three children, a distal ileostomy was also used. The patients and their parents were taught to use the gastrostomy as a vent whenever distention, pain, or vomiting developed. Some patients required daily venting, whereas others used the enterostomy as a vent only during obstructive episodes.

Results

After the initiation of TPN and a venting gastrostomy, 12 of the 17 children required no further hospital admissions for intestinal obstruction. Five of the patients were admitted for obstruction, a total of 11 times. Thus, once the 17 patients were given TPN and had received a venting gastrostomy, they required only 11 hospital admissions for obstruction in a total of 89 patient-years, or 0.12 admissions per patient-year. In comparison, prior to TPN and enterostomy treatment, these same patients required 44 admissions for obstruction in a total of approximately 36 patient-years, or 1.22 admissions per patient-year. Moreover, following placement of the venting gastrostomy only three laparotomies for obstructive problems were performed in two children.

During the course of treatment, two children died. Only one of these deaths may be attributed to the pseudo-obstruction or its treatment. This 2-year-old child who had been maintained on TPN since birth, and who had received a gastrostomy when she was 6 days old, died from aspiration pneumonia complicated by central venous catheter sepsis. None of 15 children with gastrostomies had tube-related complications. Problems related to the TPN catheter, however, were seen more frequently. Seven children required hospitalization at some point for either sepsis, thrombosis, or other catheter-related complications.

Discussion

Chronic intestinal pseudo-obstruction is a clinical syndrome in which the signs and symptoms of intestinal obstruction are present, but no mechanical obstructing lesions exists (Golladay and Byrne 1981; Shuffler 1981). Although this condition is rare, an unusually large number of therapeutic modalities have been recommended for treatment. None of these suggested remedies has been particularly effective, including elemental diets, antibiotics, steroids, indomethacin, various hormones, prostaglandins, and resective or bypass surgery (Golladay and Byrne 1981). More recently, several authors (Byrne et al. 1977; Shaw et al. 1979; Greenall and Gough 1983) have suggested that children with the most severe forms of chronic intestinal pseudo-obstruction may be treated with long-term TPN. The long-term results of this form of therapy have not yet been determined. The present study on 17 children with chronic intestinal pseudo-obstruction lends support to this method of treatment. Although various bypass and resective operations have been suggested for children with well-defined anatomic patterns of pseudo-obstruction, most authorities now recommend avoidance of laparotomy (Golladay and Byrne 1981; Shuffler 1981; Shaw et al. 1979; Shuffler and Deitch 1980).

The present study is the first to report a large number of children with pseudo-obstruction in whom a venting gastrostomy has been part of the management. The rationale for the gastrostomy is to spare these children the frequent need for nasogastric intubation and repetitive hospitalizations for obstruction. Even through nutrition is maintained with parenteral nutrition, these patients are encouraged to eat when they are feeling well. When they develop symptoms, however, they merely drain the gastrostomy while at home, both to relieve pain and distention and to avoid vomiting and hospitalization. That this method of therapy is effective is reflected by the fact that the number of hospitalizations per patient-year was reduced by more than sixfold after the addition of TPN and placement of a venting gastrostomy.

A small intestinal biopsy should also be performed at the time of laparotomy and gastrostomy placement. Children with intestinal pseudo-obstruction characteristically have low-amplitude primary peristaltic contractions, disordered distal peristalsis, and diminished lower esophageal sphincter pressures. Sullivan and his associates (Sullivan et al. 1977) have determined that intestinal smooth-muscle slow-wave activity, as well as spike and motor responses to exogenous neurohormonal stimulation, are intact.

As has been indicated by Byrne and associates (Byrne et al. 1981), the roentgenographic hallmarks of chronic intestinal pseudo-obstruction are (a) absence of stricture, (b) absent, decreased, or disorganized intestinal motility, (c) dilated loops of small intestines, including the proximal duodenum, and (d) decreased or absent haustral markings and/or redundancies of the colon. The histologic criteria for establishment of the diagnosis of chronic intestinal pseudo-obstruction remains controversial. Whereas some investigators have reported normal histologic features, others have noted pathologic changes in the neuroarchitecture, smooth muscle, or both. Shuffler and Jonak (1982) have stressed that pathologic lesions of intestinal neuropathy can be missed by conventional light microscopy and may be apparent only when a silver technique is used to visualize the myenteric plexus. It has also been suggested that chronic pseudo-obstruction may have multiple causes and, therefore, different pathologic findings.

References

Byrne WJ, Cipell L, Euler AR, et al (1977) Chronic idiopathic intestinal pseudo-obstruction syndrome in children: clinical characteristics and prognosis. J Pediatr 90:585-589

Byrne WJ, Cipell L, Ament ME, et al (1981) Chronic idiopathic intestinal pseudo-obstruction syndrome: radiologic signs in children with emphasis on differentiation from mechanical obstruction. Diagn Imag 50:294-304

Golladay ES, Byrne WJ (1981) Intestinal pseudo-obstruction. Surg Gynecol Obstet 153:257-273

Greenall MJ, Gough MH (1983) Chronic idiopathic intestinal pseudo-obstruction in infancy and its successful treatment with parenteral feeding. Dis Colon Rectum 26:53-54

Shaw A, Shaffer H, Teja K, et al (1979) A perspective for pediatric surgeons: chronic idiopathic intestinal pseudo-obstruction. J Pediatr Surg 14:719-727

Shuffler MD (1981) Causes of chronic idiopathic intestinal pseudo-obstruction syndromes. Med Clin North Am 65:1332-1358

Shuffler MD, Deitch EA (1980) Chronic idiopathic intestinal pseudo-obstruction: a surgical approach. Ann Surg 192:752-761

Shuffler MD, Jonak Z (1982) Chronic idiopathic intestinal pseudo-obstruction caused by a degenerative disorder of the myenteric plexus: the use of Smith's method to define the neuropathology. Gastroenterology 82:476-486

Sullivan MA, Snape WJ Jr, Matarazzo SA, et al (1977) Gastrointestinal myoelectrical activity in idiopathic intestinal pseudo-obstruction. N Engl J Med 297:233-238

The Importance of Oral Sodium Replacement in Ileostomy Patients

P. Sacher[1], J. Hirsig[1], J. Gresser[1], and L. Spitz[2]

Summary

The main function of the colon is fluid and sodium conservation. In ileostomy patients these colonic functions are lacking. The consequence is excessive loss of fluid and sodium, failure to thrive, and skin excoriation around the ileostomy. Patients with ileostomies require 6–10 mmol/kg sodium per day. With ordinary feeds, infants receive 2–4 mmol/kg sodium; therefore the sodium deficit may be estimated at 4–6 mmol/kg per day. Monitoring of adequate sodium substitution is best carried out by measuring the concentration of sodium in spot urine. Levels higher than 10 mmol/l sodium signify an adequate oral sodium intake. During the initial period of oral feeding, glucose excretion in the ileostomy fluid must be monitored, as glucose-positive ileostomy effluence necessitates additional sodium substitution in order to activate the sodium and glucose cotransport. Thirty neonates with ileostomies were followed-up retrospectively. All patients received a sodium substitution of at least 4–6 mmol/kg orally per day. The 30 patients had a total of 4769 ileostomy-days. All patients were successfully fed orally and most of them nursed at home until closure of the ileostomy.

Zusammenfassung

Das Kolon spielt eine entscheidende Rolle im Wasser- und Elektrolythaushalt. Durch das Anlegen einer Ileostomie werden diese Funktionen des Kolons ausgeschaltet. Dies führt zu einem massiven Wasser- und Natriumverlust, Entwicklungsstörungen und oft zu enormen Hautproblemen im Bereich des Ileostomas. Der Na-Bedarf von Ileostomiepatienten liegt bei 6–10 mmol/kg KG/Tag. Die Na-Zufuhr mit normaler Ernährung beträgt 2–4 mmol/kg KG/Tag, so daß Ileostomiepatienten ein Na-Defizit von ca. 4–6 mmol/kg KG/Tag aufweisen, das entsprechend substituiert werden muß. Die Na-Substitution kann durch Messung des Na-Gehalts in einer Urinportion überwacht werden. Werte über 10 mmol/l bedeuten eine genügende Substitution. Während des enteralen Ernährungsaufbaues soll auch die Glukoseausscheidung in der Ileostomieflüssigkeit gemessen werden, da auch bei positivem Glukosenachweis im Stuhl die Na-Substitution erhöht werden muß, um die Glukoseresorption über die Natrium-Glukose-Pumpe wieder zu aktivieren. Es wird über 30 Neugeborene mit Ileostomien berichtet. Alle Patienten erhielten eine Na-Substitution von mindestens 4–6 mmol/kg KG/Tag peroral. Die 30 Patienten weisen zusammen 4769 Ileostomietage auf, was einem Zeitraum von ca. 13 Jahren entspricht. Alle Patienten konnten bis zum Enterostomieverschluß normal ernährt und die meisten zu Hause von den Eltern gepflegt werden. Die Patienten zeigten eine gute Gewichtszunahme.

Résumé

La fonction principale du côlon est la conservation d'eau et d'électrolytes. En effectuant une iléostomie, les fonctions du côlon sont interrompues. La conséquence est une perte massive d'eau

---

[1] University Children's Hospital, Steinwiesstr. 75, CH-8032 Zurich, Switzerland
[2] Hospital for Sick Children, Great Ormond Street, London, UK

et de sodium, un mauvais développement et des problèmes de peau autour de l'iléostoma. Le besoin en sodium des opérés s'élève de 6 à 10 mmol/kg/jour. Une alimentation normale apporte 2 à 4 mmol/kg/jour, ce qui mène à un déficit de sodium de 4 à 6 mmol/kg/jour pour les opérés, un déficit qui doit être substitué en conséquence. La substitution de sodium peut être contrôlée par la mesuration du contenu de sodium dans une portion d'urine. Des valeurs de 10 mmol/l et plus signalent une substitution suffisante. Pendant la période initiale de l'alimentation orale, il est conseillé de contrôler la sécrétion de glucose dans le liquide de l'iléostoma, puisque la substitution de sodium doit être augmentée lors de preuves positives de glucose dans la selle pour réactiver la résorption de glucose par la pompe de sodium-glucose.

Nous rapportons sur 30 nouveau-nés avec iléostomie. Tous les opérés ont reçu une substitution de sodium d'au moins 4 à 6 mmol/kg/jour par voie orale. Les 30 malades représentent un total de 4769 jours d'iléostomie, ce qui correspond à une période de 13 années. Tous les malades ont été nourris normalement et la plupart a été soignée à domicile par les parents jusqu'à la fermeture de l'iléostomie. L'augmentation de poids a été satisfaisante chez tous les patients.

An ileostomy is often a life-saving first-stage procedure in neonatal intestinal diseases such as necrotizing enterocolitis (NEC) and total colonic aganglionosis. In infants, however, the procedure has had a poor reputation due to the propensity to fluid and electrolyte imbalance, failure to thrive, and excoriation of the skin adjacent to the stoma. The fear of an ileostomy was shared by many pediatric surgeons, as illustrated in the first edition of *Neonatal Surgery* (Rickham) in 1969, where a 56% mortality is quoted. In the 1978 edition of *Neonatal Surgery* it is stated that "it is very important not to delay closure of the enterostomy as the fluid losses through the high enterostomy can be considerable as the infant's abdominal skin will rapidly become very inflamed because of irritation by the liquid intestinal contents" (Lister and Rickham 1969). It is, however, very interesting that Gross in 1953 and Swenson in 1958 (Raffensberger 1980) in their textbooks suggest early oral feeding to prevent excessive ileostomy secretion. Gross recommends the administration of fluids such as soup and sweet and salty watery solutions in the early postoperative period.

Materials and Methods

Between January 1983 and December 1985, 22 patients had an ileostomy performed at the University Children's Hospital Zurich. Eight patients operated in 1982 at the Hospital for Sick Children, Great Ormond Street, London, have also been included in this series. All patients received supplementary sodium chloride of at least 4 mmol/kg per day. Total body sodium content was monitored by measuring the sodium excretion in spot urine. If urine sodium was below 10 mmol/l, the sodium supplement was increased. When oral nutrition was commenced, the concentration of glucose in the ileostomy fluid was measured by clinitest. When clinitest was positive, sodium supplement was increased.

Table 1. Patients with ileostomies

Patient	Sex	Gestation (weeks)	Birth weight		Diagnosis	Ileostomy			Ileostomy closure		
			Kg	Percentile		Age (days)	Weight	Percentile	Time elapse (days)	Weight	Percentile
1. K.R.	M	36	1800	<3	NEC	5	1800	<3	373	8900	10–25
2. L.C.	M	35	1200	<3	NEC	25	1200	<3	90	4000	3–10
3. M.B.	F	36	1380	<3	NEC	20	1300	<3	93	4000	10–25
4. D.V.	M	32	900	<3	NEC	10	900	<3	62	2000	3
5. S.B.	M	36	1750	<3	NEC	40	1750	<3	206	6400	25–50
6. M.S.	M	39	3760	50–90	HD	2	3760	50–90	510	10500	25–50
7. S.H.	M	40	3400	50	HD	12	3400	50	272	7500	10
8. M.L.	F	40	2800	10	HD	5	2800	10	304	5800	<3
9. W.R.	M	30	890	<3	NEC	18	1130	<3	140	4030	10–50
10. B.F.	F	40	3350	50	HD	150	5740	50	270	9180	50
11. L.R.	M	39	3700	90	NEC	8	3600	90	70	4400	3
12. W.B.	M	40	3000	10–50	NEC	7	2900	10–50	72	4900	10
13. H.N.	F	40	3500	50–90	MP	120	4060	<3	550	11300	50
14. G.	M	37	2780	90	NEC	9	2780	90	230	5500	3
15. G.J.	M	31	1380	10–50	NEC	5	1200	10–50	155	4710	75–90
16. R.M.	M	41	3560	50	NEC	8	3600	50	110	7000	75–90
17. B.S.	M	28	1180	50	NEC	21	1340	10	210	4700	3
18. R.C.	M	39	2860	10	NEC	4	2710	10	90	4680	10–25
19. T.J.	F	31	3640	>90	MP	1	2660	>90	83	2920	10
20. P.A.	M	40	4120	90	HD	33	4640	90	160	8510	>90
21. K.S.	M	37	3000	50	HD	151	7400	75	282	8020	<3
22. P.R.	M	40	4200	>90	IP	16	4190	90	60	5100	90
23. B.H.	M	40	2980	10–50	NEC	7	3150	10–50	72	4990	50
24. K.G.	F	38	2780	50	NEC	5	2360	50	32	3190	10
25. S.K.	M	37	2200	10	NEC	3	2500	3	–	–	–
26. W.S.	F	34	1730	10–50	NEC	5	1970	10–50	–	–	–
27. B.M.	F	40	2640	10	IA	3	2320	10	60	4170	10–50
28. W.M.	F	39	3215	50	MI	1	3290	50	96	3800	3
29. B.R.	M	38	3000	50	Omph.	7	3240	50	103	5700	97
30. K.F.	F	40	3500	50	NEC	20	3760	50	26	3800	50

NEC, Necrotizing enterocolitis; HD, Hirschsprung's disease; MP, meconium peritonitis; IP, ileal perforation; IA, ileal atresia; MI, meconium ileus; Omph., omphalocele

Table 2. Indications for ileostomy in 30 patients

Indication	Number of patients
Necrotizing enterocolitis	18
Hirschsprung's disease	6
Meconium peritonitis	2
Meconium ileus	1
Ileal perforation	1
Ileal atresia	1
Omphalocele	1

Results

The results are summarized in Table 1. There were 20 boys and 10 girls in the series, of whom ten were preterm infants. Birth weight was below the 3rd percentile in six cases. The distribution of indications for ileostomy are shown in Table 2. Seven patients had a weight below the 3rd percentile at the time of ileostomy. Two of the 30 patients (cases 25, 26), operated on for perforated NEC, died of septicemia, one on the day of operation and the second on the 17th postoperative day. Total ileostomy-days amounted to 4769 — equivalent to almost 13 years. With an oral sodium supplement of 4–20 mmol/kg per 24 h it was possible to feed all ten patients orally, and most of them have been nursed at home by their parents. Three patients (cases 14, 17, 30) developed complications. The first had recurrent episodes of contaminated small bowel syndrome (CSBS). The second also had a CSBS due to a stenosing stoma following a peristomal abscess. The third patient developed an osmotic dyspepsia despite adequate sodium supplement when formula milk was introduced. Since the condition improved when feeds were changed to an elementary diet, the most probable cause of diarrhea was a transitory deficiency of disaccharidase. At the time of closure of the enterostomy only two patients were below the 3rd percentile. Three patients still have their ileostomies. In 25 patients the enterostomy has been closed. There were no late deaths in this series.

Discussion

To diminish the excessive loss of fluids and electrolytes in ileostomy patients, numerous procedures have been advocated. Some authors recommend delaying intestinal motility either with operations such as reversed segments or pharmacologically with loperamide. H_2 blocking substances have also been suggested. Prostaglandin synthetase blocking agents to reduce intestinal secretion are a further possibility. Codeine phosphate and mechanical blockage by balloon have been recommended. No single procedure was reliable in simplifying the management of ileostomies in infants.

Referring to the physiology of the colon, which consists mainly of sodium and water reabsorption, it seems logical that the ileostomy patient with exclusion of the colon would be prone to excessive loss of fluids and electrolytes with consecutive severe metabolic complications. That the ileum gradually adopts colonic functions such as the reabsorption of sodium and water was studied in 1972 by Ricour et al. (1973). They found a very limited ability of the ileum for sodium conservation. The requirements of sodium in patients with an ileostomy may be as high as 6–10 mmol/kg per day. The mean sodium intake by breast milk, formula milk, and elementary diet is 2–4 mmol/kg per day. Therefore, patients with an ileostomy need a sodium supplement of 4–6 mmol/kg per day. Progressive sodium depletion not only leads to imbalance of fluids and electrolytes but also provokes a general metabolic catastrophe. Insufficient sodium concentrations within the lumen of the bowel result in ineffective absorption of glucose due to failure of the cotransport of sodium and glucose (Bell et al. 1980). Despite the deficiency of calory intake there is an osmotic diarrhea.

The sodium supplement must be controlled by measuring the sodium concentrations in the 24-h urine, as hyponatremia occurs only later due to the defective sodium homostasis. Therefore, in infants with an ileostomy, urinary sodium excretion is a more sensitive gauge of sodium homostasis than is serum sodium concentration. Schwarz et al. (1983) found a high correlation of sodium concentration in spot urine and the value of a 24-h collection. They showed that sodium concentration in spot urine is a simple and reliable indicator of sodium depletion. Values of more than 10 mmol/l in the absence of adrenal or renal disease or diuretics provide reassurance of sufficient sodium supplement. Clinical correlation is mandatory to determine the need for additional supplement when lower values are found because the urine sodium concentration of healthy growing infants is often less than 10 mmol/l.

According to Hill et al. (1975), measurement of the sodium/potassium ratio in the ileostomy fluid and the urine permits an even more precise monitoring of sodium homostasis. Sufficient sodium supplement is achieved when values are less than 15 and more than 1. Some of our children needed a much higher dose of sodium than recommended by Ricour et al. (1973) to prevent excessive loss of fluid. When feeding is initiated, the glucose concentration in the ileostomy fluid should also be measured, as sodium supplement needs to be augmented when glucose concentrations are high in order to activate the cotransport of sodium and glucose. The cause of high concentrations of glucose in the ileostomy fluid is more often due to an insufficient sodium supplement than a deficiency of disaccharidase.

In cases of salt-losing ileostomy diarrhea despite adequate oral saline supplement, administration of an oral glucose electrolyte mixture (e.g., Elotrans, Oralpedon) is effective in restoring the sodium balance (Ward et al. 1984).

References

Bell GH, Emslie-Smith D, Paterson C (1980) Digestion and absorption in the intestine. In: Bell GH (ed) Textbook of physiology, 10th edn. Churchill Livingstone, Edinburgh, pp 76–77

Gross RE (1953) The surgery of infancy and childhood. Saunders, Philadelphia

Hill GL, Mair WS, Goligher JC (1975) Cause and management of high volume output salt-depleting ileostomy. Br J Surg 62:720–726

Lister J, Rickham PP (1978) Necrotizing enterocolitis; bacterial and meconium peritonitis. In: Rickham PP, Lister J, Irving I (eds) Neonatal surgery, 2nd edn. Butterworths, London, p 419

Raffensberger JG (1980) Swenson's pediatric surgery. Appleton-Century-Crofts, New York

Rickham PP (1969) Meconium and bacterial peritonitis. In: Rickham PP, Johnston JH (eds) Neonatal surgery. Butterworths, London, p 361

Rickham PP, Johnston JH (eds) (1969) Neonatal surgery. Butterworths, London

Ricour C, Millot M, Balsan S (1973) Sodium conservation after total or subtotal colonic resection in children. Scand J Gastroenterol 8:743–750

Schwarz KB, Ternberg JL, Bell MJ, et al (1983) Sodium needs of infants and children with ileostomy. J Pediatr 102:509–513

Ward K, Murray B, Neale G, et al (1984) Treatment of salt-losing ileostomy diarrhea with an oral glucose polymer electrolyte solution. Ir J Med Sci 153:77–78

Subject Index

abnormal bowel function (s. rectoanal reflex)
adapatation reaction 143, 147
adynamic bowel syndrome (s. bowel syndrome)
aganglionosis, segmental 179
anal canal 90
– –, contractions 44
– –, length 80, 81
– –, pressure 46, 61, 108, 109
– –, relaxation 98, 102
– pressure, maximal 100, 102
anomalies, high-type 34
–, intermediate-type 34
–, low-type 34
anorectal function 71, 72
– length 147
– malformations 23, 33, 116
– –, classification 34
– –, clinical assessment 116
– –, manometric study 116
– –, resting pressure 117
– manometry 21, 40, 43, 49, 59, 61, 68, 79, 80, 88, 100, 108, 204
– –, computer system 23
– –, computerized analysis 21
– –, development 143
– –, limitation 145
– –, practical significance 142
– –, pressure-recording system 22
– –, scientific significance 153
– motility 77
– pressure profile 147, 148
– reflex 71, 73, 118, 119
– structures, manometric study 118
anorectum, motility 67, 73
anus, imperforate (s. imperforate)

bacterial overgrowth, secondary pseudo-obstruction 136
balloon distension 45
– – method 42
bowel obstruction 53, 165
– –, mechanical 135
– syndrome, adynamic 138, 194
– –, short 135

Chagas' disease 135
chronic idiopathic intestinal pseudo-obstruction (CIIP – s. pseudo-obstruction)
colon atresia 53
– inertia 203
– polyp 23
–, transient functional obstruction 202, 203
–, – – –, biopsy 202
–, – – –, development 202
–, – – –, manometry 202
colonic aganglionosis, total 217, 218, 227
– –, –, late complication, fistulae 218
– dysmotility 177
– haustration 159
– motility 155, 159
– obstruction (CO) 207
– stenosis 54
colonic ultrasonography
    (s. ultrasonography)
colostomy 54
computerized analysis 23
– –, image processing 24
– –, – analysis 25
congenital megacolon 205
constipation 50, 51, 54, 62, 71, 89
–, chronic 23, 25, 162
contamined small bowel syndrome (CSBS) 166
continence 62, 86, 147
–, evaluation 149
–, partial 147
–, reaction 144, 147
–, score 152
constractions 127
CSBS
    (s. contamined small bowel syndrome)

defecation 72, 89
–, clinical assessment 99
–, induction 145
defecogram 111, 112
defecography 108, 111
diabetic enteropathy 134
diarrhea, bacterial 133

Subject Index

electrical activity   126, 138
– contraction complex   131
– control activity (ECA)   127
– response activity (ERA)   127
electromechanical rhythm   127
electromyographic examination   33
enteric nervous system, development   173, 181
enterocolitis   138
–, necrotizing (NEC)   54, 227, 229
external sphincter contraction, active   147
– – –, duration   147
– – muscle   33
– – –, development   37
– – – score   36
– –, relaxation   98, 102

fecal continence   60, 62, 110
– retention   149
fibrosis, intestinal wall (s. intestinal wall)
fistulae   219

haustral contractions   159
high-pressure zone   108
Hirschsprung's disease   7, 10, 23, 28, 43, 50, 54, 59, 68, 77, 137, 148, 163, 179, 181, 217, 228
– –, anorectal function   72
– –, – motility   77
– –, diagnosis   40, 49
– –, pseudo   203
hyperganglionosis   179
hyperthyrosis   132
hypoganglionosis   179, 214
hypothyrosis   132

Ikeda's z-shaped anastomosis   59
ileal atresia   229
– perforation   229
ileocecal valve   156, 157, 159
– region   159
ileostomy   226
–, indications   229
image analysis   23
immaturity, functional   203
imperforate anus   7, 10, 86
– –, postoperative continence   115
– –, rectoanal pressure studies   115
incontinence   62, 63, 73, 89, 147
–, constipation   150, 15
–, myogenic   151
–, neurogenic   151
infusion open-tip method   79
internal anal sphincter muscle, electrical activity   131

–, sphincter, performance   144
– –, relaxation   144, 147
intestinal idiopathic pseudo-obstruction   136
– motility   126
– –, disturbances   132
– obstruction, functional, newborn   203
– wall, fibrosis   193

manometry (s. anorectal manometry)
mass contractions   149, 159
– –, propulsive   161
maturation, disturbance   214
meconium ileus   53, 229
– peritonitis   229
– plug syndrome   203
MEN (s. multiple endocrine neoplasia)
meningocele   50, 54
migrating motor complex (MMC)   127
– – –, interdigestive   134
– – –, –, disturbances   134
motility disorders, innervation-related   173
– disturbances, electrophysiological principles   125
– malfunction   193
multiple endocrine neoplasia (MEN)   189
myectomy (s. rectal myectomy)
myelomeningocele   23

NEC (s. enterocolitis)
neuronal intestinal dysplasia (NID)   155, 186
– –, classification   189
– – –, clinical feature   188
newborn, functional intestinal obstruction (s. intestinal)
nicotine uptake   134
NID (s. neuronal intestinal dysplasia)

omphalocele   229
oral sodium replacement   226
osteomyelitis, sacral   219

peristaltic activity   151
postoperative bowel atonia   135
pressure changes   70
– probes   22
– profile   147, 205, 206
– sensor probe   7
– vector   25, 30
– – analysis   30
– volume curves   92, 93
propulsive contraction   162, 163
pseudo-obstruction   177, 179
– –, chronic idiopathic intestinal (CIIP)   188, 194
– –, – intestinal, surgical management   221

Subject Index

psychic stress   134
pyloric stenosis, hypertrophic   175

radial variation analysis   24, 30
rectal atresia   53
– compliance   92, 93, 108
– maturation   145
– motility   159
– myectomy   77, 78, 81
– pressure   61, 108
– prolapse, anorectal motility   105
– –, operation   107
– segmentation   162
– sensation   71, 72
– stenosis   50, 54
– stimulation   51, 68
rectoanal reflex   5, 7, 10, 50, 51, 54, 56, 68, 69, 70, 80, 81, 108, 109
– –, abnormal bowel function   9, 50
– –, analysis   53
– –, clinical studies   7
– –, corrective surgery   83
– –, experimental studies   12
– –, inhibitory   25, 101
– –, neuronal control   5
– –, postoperative cases   10
– relaxation reflex   42, 43, 44, 46, 60, 61, 62, 63
– response   14
reflex anorectal pressure, profile   91, 92
– pressure profile   86
relaxation reflex   147
resting pressure   61, 62, 205
– –, anal canal   80, 81
– –, contractions   42
– –, profile   79, 80, 81, 82, 110
– –, rectum   80, 81
rhythmic contractions   108
– –, frequency   62
– wave, basal   82
– – contractions, frequency   61
– –, frequency   70

sclerodermia, secondary pseudo-obstruction   136
short bowel syndrome (s. bowel syndrome)

sigmoid, segmental dilatation   53
slow waves   127, 131, 137
– –, disturbances   131
– –, low-frequency   138
small bowel contamination   165
– – dysmotility   176
– – obstruction   167
– – syndrome (s. contamined)
– intestine, volvulus   53
– left colon syndrome (SLC)   207
– – – –, neonatal   203
Soave-Denda operation   67
soiling   62, 63
sphincter muscle (s. external sphincter muscle)
sphincter relaxation   52
–, internal   12
spike activity, disturbances   133, 134
– bursts, short   131
– –, long   131
– potential bursts   127
spikes   127
spina bifida
– –, anorectal pressure profile   101, 102
– –, – – –, patterns   98, 99
– –, clinical assessment of defecation   101, 102
– –, management of defecation   97
– –, maximal anal pressure   100, 102
– –, rectoanal inhibitory reflex   101, 102
sqeeze pressure   147, 148
staining   73
static pressure, maximum   90
– –, mean   90
Sudeck's operation   107

thyroid, aplasia   50, 53, 54

ultrasonographic examination   113
ultrasonographic, colonic   155
–, –, technique   159

vagotomy   134
vomiting   133

wall contractions, concentric   159
water-filled open-tip method   61

Progress in Pediatric Surgery

Springer-Verlag Berlin
Heidelberg New York London
Paris Tokyo Hong Kong

Volume 23

L. Spitz, London; P. Wurnig, Vienna;
T. A. Angerpointner, Munich (Eds.)

Surgery in Solitary Kidney and Corrections of Urinary Transport Disturbances

1989. VIII, 205 pp. 136 figs. 34 tabs.
Hardcover ISBN 3-540-50485-0

Volume 23 deals with selected topics of pediatric urology and problems of malformed external genitalia. Pathophysiology, diagnosis, treatment and outcome in solitary kidneys and other severe malformations of the urinary tract are described by internationally appreciated authors. Severe malformations of the anogenital region, such as cloacal malformations, congenital adrenal hyperplasia, epispadias and hypospadias are the great challenge to pediatric surgery. New insights, techniques and alternative methods are discussed in the second part of this volume to give the reader a review of the state art in this field.

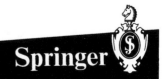

Progress in Pediatric Surgery

Volume 22
L. Spitz, London; P. Wurnig, Vienna; T. A. Angerpointner, Munich (Eds.)

Pediatric Surgical Oncology

1989. VIII, 180 pp. 78 figs. 44 tabs. Hardcover
ISBN 3-540-17769-8

Volume 21
P. Wurnig, Vienna (Ed.)

Trachea and Lung Surgery in Childhood

1987. X, 147 pp. 75 figs. Hardcover
ISBN 3-540-17232-7

Volume 20
P. P. Rickham, Zurich (Ed.)

Historical Aspects of Pediatric Surgery

1986. X, 285 pp. 119 figs. Hardcover
ISBN 3-540-15960-6

Volume 19
P. Wurnig, Vienna (Ed.)

Long-gap Esophageal Atresia Prenatal Diagnosis of Congenital Malformations

1986. XII, 205 pp. 86 figs. Hardcover
ISBN 3-540-15881-2

Springer-Verlag Berlin
Heidelberg New York London
Paris Tokyo Hong Kong

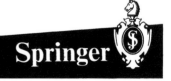

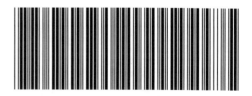